Natural Medicine and Herbal Remedies for Preppers

Survival Secrets of Wilderness Wellness

Carlos Mack

Table of Contents

EXTRA BONUS

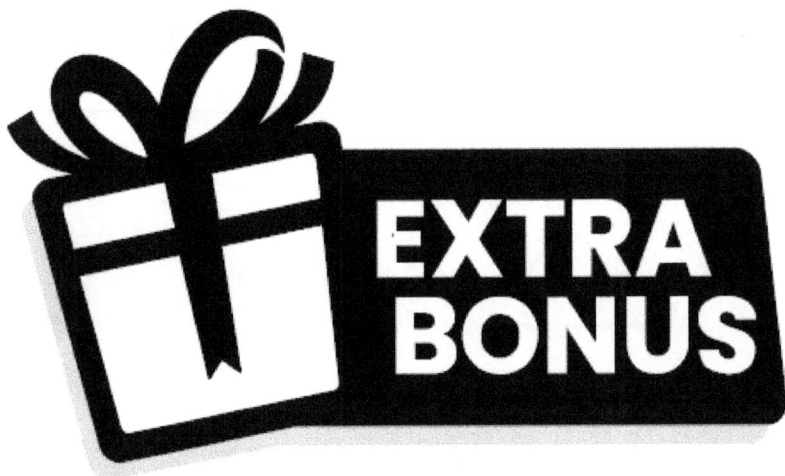

Thank you for embarking on this literary journey with me! Your support and enthusiasm for my book mean the world. As a token of gratitude, I'm thrilled to offer you exclusive access to the "Herbal Medicine Starter Guide." Simply scan the QR code below and drop your email to receive this invaluable tool – no strings attached, just a little something extra for being a loyal reader. Your continued support is truly appreciated, and I hope this bonus enriches your prepping journey in the most extraordinary ways!

⬇ SCAN THE QR CODE BELOW ⬇

SCAN ME

Introduction

My friend Ray Franklin wrestled with relentless heartburn for years, exhausting every over-the-counter remedy available without relief. He was intimately familiar with nearly every antacid brand, investing a small fortune in these attempts to ease his pain. Eventually, Ray lost hope of finding a solution. Then, one day while browsing the internet, he stumbled upon articles about ulcer home remedies. Among the search results were two transformative pieces—one detailing how to create fermented cabbage juice for ulcers and another advocating ginger juice among various remedies.

Since discovering these natural solutions, Ray hasn't spent a penny or endured sleepless nights. He now enjoys foods previously forbidden by his ulcer and feels liberated from its grip. Today, Ray harbors deep skepticism toward pharmaceutical companies producing antacids, convinced they deliberately overlook superior and more affordable natural alternatives. Ray's experience has convinced him that not only heartburn but every illness has a more economical and effective natural remedy waiting to be discovered!

Numerous individuals grapple with illnesses despite exploring various treatments that often prove ineffective. Whether due to inadequate medications or financial constraints, many face these hurdles. Rest assured that a cost-effective, natural remedy is waiting to be discovered if you find yourself in this situation. All it requires is a sincere search. This book serves as your guide toward finding that solution. Sometimes the solution is even in your backyard, nearby shrubs, a local vegetable market, or a garden. The challenge for most people, including preppers, is figuring out which herbs to use, how to get them, what the preparation steps are, and how to store them for a long time without spoilage.

Uncovering the herbal remedies for your ailment might make you wish you'd discovered them sooner, potentially saving you years or months of pain and expenses. Whether cultivating them in your garden, purchasing them online or foraging, accessing these herbs is straightforward.

Crafting delightful juices, teas, or recipes from these herbs is both simple and gratifying. You can convert herbs for external use into ointments, inhalants, gels, infusions, or soaps. This comprehensive guidebook provides you with the knowledge to execute these processes and create personalized herbal formulas that are perfectly tailored to your health requirements and easy to incorporate into your routine.

When your medicines are customized to smell and taste exactly as you prefer, undergoing treatment with herbs will hardly feel like one. Crucially, this tailored approach eliminates the need for spending huge amounts on pharmaceutical drugs and sidestepping their potential side effects. Bid farewell to frequent hospital visits, waiting room queues, and the challenge of swallowing unpleasant pills and syrups. Countless individuals have seamlessly adopted this method, and you can effortlessly join their ranks as well.

It would be a mistake not to learn about potential herbal solutions to your health problems and general wellness. Disasters and financial crises happen to people more often than ever, and you may not always find a doctor. Knowing the herbs that will cure you and keep you healthy is a priceless skill in today's world. Ancient people didn't have pharmaceutical drugs but lived healthy lives. Many herbalists rely completely on plants as their primary medicine but are very healthy. Herbal therapy is generally accepted by governments and higher institutions rather than being denounced.

Without the proper guide, wannabe herbal enthusiasts may try to adopt herbalism the wrong way, leading to less benefit or even harm. Understanding the principles of herbalism and how to integrate herbs into your life is critical to forging the deep human-plant connection necessary to benefit from herbs and navigate the associated risks. Adapting to herbs can take time, especially with less-than-perfect planning. Zero or inadequate planning is the reason newbies struggle with the transition from conventional to botanical medicine. By taking a few basic steps, you can simplify and speed up the process and avoid the risks that come with some herbs.

Why should you heed my words? What qualifies me as an authority on herbal remedies and natural survival techniques? For years, I've immersed myself in the world of preparation, drawing from extensive research and hands-on experience to craft comprehensive, practical guides. My expertise isn't rooted in stoking fear but in genuinely empowering families like yours to navigate crises with resilience. This book marks my fourth in the realm of preparation and survival. The previous three have all achieved the coveted #1 new release badge on Amazon. Am I a survival expert? As I've stated all along, I firmly believe that claiming expertise imposes limits; there's an infinite well of knowledge to explore. However, I do declare an unwavering passion for preparation and an unquenchable thirst for ongoing learning. I'm here to be your companion on this journey toward your green pharmacy revolution!

This book begins with a two-paragraph story of a lone Syrian refugee who might have died if not for the herbal know-how of a local shepherd. It highlights some shocking statistics and facts about the dangerous state of our world and why we should prepare for potential future disasters. You'll learn a brief history of herbalism and the challenges and stages it passed through.

Uncover over 90 herbs, each detailed with their uses, dosage, and vital information. This exhaustive research distinguishes this book as your ultimate reference guide, setting it apart from the rest by providing comprehensive insights into these herbs. There's also an in-depth guide on buying, foraging, and gardening herbs. Finally, you'll know how to create herbal remedies, store them, and integrate them into your lifestyle in the safest way possible.

Embark on a transformative journey through the pages ahead, where ancient wisdom meets modern necessity, equipping you with the tools to harness the power of herbs for a resilient and healthier future.

Let's go and explore friends!

Chapter 1:

Prepping and Sustainability—

Exploring Nature's Path Beyond

Survival

All survival situations revolve around a host of variables... Always adapt, think positive, and move forward. –Cody Lundin

Amir Hassan escaped with only the clothes and shoes he wore that day, plus a small gym bag containing several cans of water and a pack of biscuits. There was nothing he could do for his father and brothers now. They were all dead—shot on the same day by ISIS gunmen. Amir was the only one in the family who managed to escape. His number one goal now was to make it to the Bab Al-Hawa border crossing and into Turkiye. So far, he has covered about 10 miles on foot, with less than 3 miles left between him and the crossing.

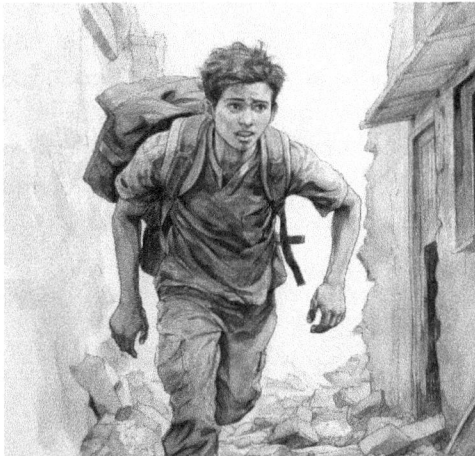

But there was a problem. His ulcers were beginning to burn, and the only edible item left in his bag was a 25-ounce bottle of water. Hassan was far from the highway, and although he saw many plants on his way, including ginger, he began to wonder whether this pain would let him reach safety. He felt his energy depleting rapidly, and he feared he would faint at any moment. After a couple of hundred yards more, he slumped into a heap of grass, slowly took out the water bottle, and drank thirstily.

Despite rehydrating and resting for over thirty minutes, he was still too weak to move. Fortunately, a shepherd, who was also headed for Bab Al-Hawa, appeared behind him. Hassan was glad to have company. After exchanging greetings, he promptly told the shepherd about his pain. Hassan described the pain to his companion, who listened keenly, after which the shepherd uprooted several ginger plants right beside Hassan. He peeled the ginger rhizomes with a knife and gave Hassan two thumb-sized rhizomes to chew and swallow the juice. Half an hour later, Amir was fit to move again, and the two continued their journey towards Bab Al-Hawa.

Anyone Could Be in Amir's Position

Armed with two decades of emergency survival wisdom, my analysis of global events and extensive research into crises and disasters have been forged through a seasoned lens. Every individual should be equipped, both physically and mentally, for the most unfavorable circumstances that the future may hold. Amidst a crisis, people may encounter sickness, injuries, hunger, and various adversities. While enduring these common tribulations, adept management and preparedness are keys to survival. It's vital to proactively address your health concerns, recognizing that support from governments, organizations, or individuals may not be consistently accessible.

The Case for Herbal Prepping

In this book, we'll focus on preparing for sickness and injuries where and when there are no doctors. It's okay that some people may reject the idea of *constant readiness* for anything that life throws at them—especially the level of preparedness I advocate for. Hence, I have to share some of my discoveries as a backup for skeptics and critics alike.

I'll just present some basic facts to you—and crucial information on the world's current situation—so you know how likely disasters are to occur and what may happen if they do. It is prudent to bear in mind that, although natural disasters exhibit a formidable force, man-made catastrophes can transcend the might exhibited by nature. They come in different forms, from economic instability to terror, from global pandemics to nuclear war, and from supply chain freezes to hurricanes.

The World's Present Situation

Anyone following current events probably knows that our world is a more dangerous place today than at any time in recent history (OUPblog, 2015). Calamities strike more often than ever before and come in different forms. Hardly would you skim 10 news headlines without discovering some shocking event. Bad things are happening in many countries—including America—with far-reaching consequences that impact the lives of many. Disasters can happen in your location and wipe out the grid along with public healthcare facilities. Here are some potential disasters that can occur in America:

War, Riot, and Domestic Strife

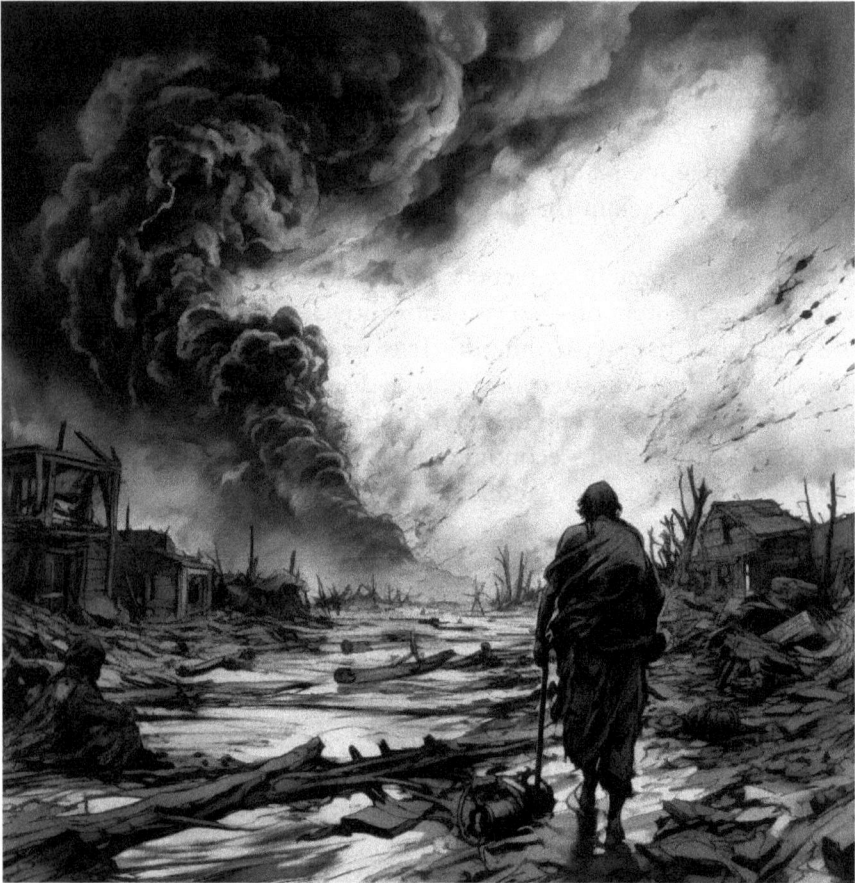

America has too many enemies to count—from individuals to organizations and countries. Washington has been avoiding large-scale foreign wars since its lesson in Iraq. It has increasingly relied on sanctions and military threats to deter enemies. But this strategy is unsustainable when you consider the rising tensions in the Middle East, Europe, and the South China Sea. Sooner or later, the US or a powerful adversary will miscalculate, dragging us into a war with no endgame in sight.

An enemy like Iran doesn't have to attack US soil to cause significant damage to our lives. Disrupting Middle Eastern oil traffic will send gas prices toward the stratosphere, with immediate repercussions on inflation worldwide (Fenton & Ghaddar, 2023). Our allied governments may collapse, taking the dollar down with them. The post-election protest of 2020 was a warning sign that America isn't immune to the kind of violent protests and riots plaguing many countries around the world today.

Biological or Chemical Terror Attack

Did you know that many individuals and organizations can acquire biological weapons? Nowadays, access to biological weapons is not limited to governments. In a survey of senior US decision-makers and policy shapers, 73% consider biological weapon attacks a major threat compared to 17% for nuclear attacks ("The Biological Weapons Threat," 2006). Do you think the government is fully prepared to handle such emergencies? COVID-19 isn't as deadly as bioweapons, but it overwhelmed America's healthcare system three years ago.

The rise of drones greatly simplifies the delivery of chemical and biological weapons over a wide area. One or more terrorists lodged in secret locations can launch coordinated attacks during a dark, rainy night. Let's assume such incidents are unlikely but possible. Are you willing to take the chance that you and your loved ones will be caught unprepared in a situation like that? Terrorists can wipe out entire families in a single attack.

Nuclear War

America has several enemies capable of launching a nuclear attack. While the chances of a large-scale attack are arguably low, the existence of these weapons and capabilities means we cannot dismiss the risks. Personally, I don't think nuclear states can indefinitely avoid an all-out nuclear war despite the reality of mutually assured destruction (MAD).

My biggest concern about the chances of a nuclear war is tactical nukes. Tactical nukes, built for conventional warfare, possess the effects of a nuclear attack. If used on a nuclear-armed adversary, the repercussions could be a tailspin toward a full-fledged nuclear war. The bottom line is that a nuclear war is possible in light of the deteriorating global order, and you should always be prepared.

EMP Attack

"A 1.4 Megaton bomb launched about 250 miles above Kansas would destroy most of the electronics that were not protected in the entire Continental United States" (*Washington State Department of Health*, 2003)

Several countries have EMP bombs, with some capable of yielding 10 megatons—almost eight times the size quoted above. According to a document published by the COMMITTEE ON OVERSIGHT AND ACCOUNTABILITY, an EMP attack that severely cripples or obliterates the US power grid can indirectly kill 90% of Americans in a prolonged power outage (Vincent, 2015). Most would die from starvation, *disease*, and societal collapse. That means most nuclear-armed countries are capable of an EMP attack (*U.S. Military Warns*, 2018).

Electricity is the lifeblood of conventional medicine. If manufacturing plants stop working, you won't get even common pills like paracetamol. This means you cannot replenish your medical supplies, which are bound to run out at some point. Only people with herbal gardens and the knowledge to use those herbs can cope healthfully for a long time. Hospitals will shut down and doctors will be hard to find. Similarly, cyberattacks can cause the same damage to electrical grids as an EMP attack (Gregory, 2023).

Natural Disasters

The National Oceanic and Atmospheric Administration has recorded as many as 122 natural disasters between 2016 and 2022, which collectively caused the deaths of 5000 people and over $1.0 trillion in damages (Workers' Rights during Natural Disasters, n.d.). Climate change contributed to many of these disasters, but the world's developed nations are reluctant to make the sacrifices required to curb climate change. It means such occurrences will be more frequent as our climate gets worse.

Some natural disasters can impact your area, such as earthquakes, floods, hurricanes, tsunamis, droughts, volcanoes, tornadoes, and many others. One of the first challenges people face during a disaster is medical aid. People will get injuries, be exposed to harsh conditions like cold, rain, and pollution, suffer violence from desperate people, and so on. The sheer number of patients usually overwhelms existing healthcare systems. This is why herbs are indispensable as a last-resort medical solution.

Climate Change Likely to Get Worse

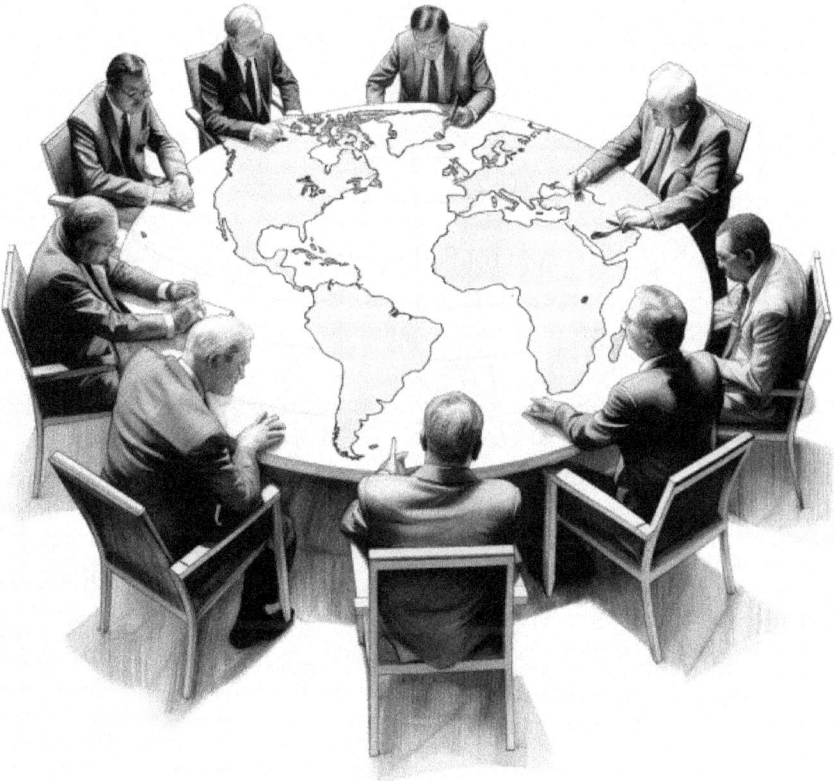

Climate change has rolled out a long list of problems for the world. From 1901 to 2020, global temperatures rose 1 °C, as a result of which natural disasters increased in frequency, scope, and intensity. Some of the problems we face from this temperature change are rising sea levels, heat waves, storms, droughts, floods, and other secondary problems these disasters lead to, such as economic disruptions, wars, and terrorism (National Oceanic and Atmospheric Administration, 2021).

The saddest news about this scary reality is that climate change looks set to get worse. It was human activity that dialed up our planet's temperature, specifically our heat- and energy-generating activities like burning fuel in machines and industries (MacMillan, 2021). For many years, developed nations have discussed limiting these activities, but they have not implemented any effective measures due to concerns that it would hinder or even reverse their economic growth. Hence, natural disasters are likely to increase and intensify. You need to prepare for them to increase your chances of survival.

Should We Prepare for Future Disasters?

So, we now know what our world is like in terms of peace and long-term security. No government or international organization can protect people perfectly or prevent wars, including the United Nations. This shouldn't be a surprise since previous generations didn't have governments that protected them from all problems. That was why they died in masse from the Black Death, Spanish Flu, Plague of Justinian, Bhola cyclone, Haiyuan earthquake, Chernobyl disaster, China floods, and more.

We have to learn from these historical catastrophes. Survival should be your #1 priority in such situations, if they happen where you live. One of the necessities is sustainable medical access. Food and shelter alone cannot handle diseases, injuries, and pains. Plant-based medicines can outlast any crisis because they are renewable and easy to produce.

How Survivors Stayed Alive With Herbs

Preparing ahead of time, or prepping, increases your chances of surviving disasters. Let's see how herbs saved the lives of many during some recent crises in India, America, and Nepal.

The Indian Tsunami of 2004

During the Indian Tsunami of 2004, rescuers used coconut water as an intravenous (IV) to rehydrate survivors in coastal communities that were cut off from medical aid and supplies. Although coconut water exits the bloodstream faster than sodium-rich IV solutions, it is better than no IV and helps a lot of survivors stay alive.

Hurricane Katrina in 2005

Hurricane Katrina killed 1,577 people in Louisiana and possibly 238 in Mississippi. After the disaster, thousands of people lacked medical assistance, including prescription drugs for pre-existing conditions. As a result, many resorted to herbal remedies like aloe vera to treat or manage burns and skin irritation, and herbal tea for digestive issues (Huelskoetter, 2015).

The Nepal Earthquake in 2015

The 2015 earthquake in Nepal killed about 90,000 people and injured another 22,000. The emergency health response was satisfactory but not complete. Subedi & Sharma (2018) treated many victims with Ayurvedic herbal tea for minor injuries.

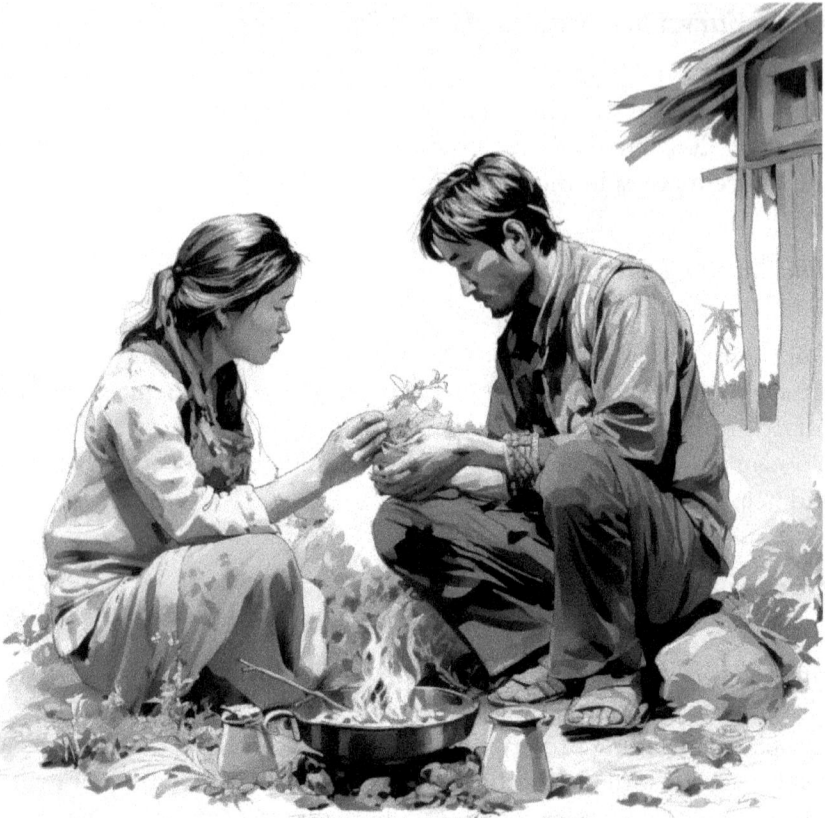

Understanding Prepping

Preparation is the act of getting yourself into a state of mental and physical preparedness to handle any future crises in order to maximize your chances of survival. The definition is simple but implementing it can be challenging for anyone who doesn't fully understand the concept or follow the right preparatory steps. To set you up for successful preparation, let's understand what it entails.

Preparedness

You are mentally and physically prepared for potential crises where you live. You will not be caught off guard by natural disasters or other calamities because you have deliberately considered the possibilities and anticipated potential outcomes, ensuring that you are fully prepared to handle any situation.

Self-Sufficiency

You've thought about and collected the basic survival items for a range of crises (ideally, the ones more likely to occur in your town or city). You aren't pinning your hopes on the government or any individual to help with food, shelter, medicine, clothing, and water.

Resilience

Preppers train their mind and body to persevere by learning and adapting in order to outlast any crises or disasters. Without resilience, your preparedness and self-sufficiency alone won't see you through certain disasters, especially if the effects are severe and last months or years.

Simply put, prepping means being *independent, adaptable,* and ready to survive any tough situation that life throws at you. But how can you *be* that if you can't personally handle your health challenges and those of your loved ones? This is why the medicinal knowledge of herbs and how to grow them is an indispensable pillar of prepping. I want to equip you with this knowledge to make your prepping flawless.

A Growing Public Awareness About Preparedness

One-third of Americans are interested in doomsday prepping. Why is that? People are realizing that the world isn't the way they thought it was. One can die at any moment if one lives unprepared. The coronavirus lockdown was brief but look how people suffered hunger and restricted medical access. Suppose it lasted a year or more. A lot of people would have died.

The survival prep industry is expected to grow at a CAGR of 7% to $2.46 billion by 2030 (Fabino, 2023). Looking at the market reports, you'll find the rapid growth isn't from selling new inventions to existing customers but from purchases by newbies and seasoned preppers. A sense of insecurity and unpreparedness tops the list of factors fueling this rapid market growth. While the report underlines Russia's war in Ukraine as a key driver, it also emphasizes other safety concerns not related to war, such as natural disasters. Three big hurricanes occurred in the US in 2017 alone (Pro, 2019b).

Off-Grid Living and the Survival Industry

Going off the grid is all-in-prepping. Some people, despite being accustomed to the comforts of modern life, remain aware of potential future calamities. The number of off-gridders in the US and Europe has doubled in the past 10 years. All these people have valid reasons for disconnecting from the grid. Some have had enough of the urban lifestyle, some want to be self-reliant, and many others did so to better their chances of surviving a catastrophe like the coronavirus.

Regardless of the reason for going off-grid, fans consider it a safer or even better way of living. There's usually a sudden leap in the number of off-gridders whenever a public disaster occurs. Due to such leaps in demand, survival prepping firms are going beyond manufacturing individual gadgets to complete survival tool sets, where preppers get everything they need in one whole package. In the United States, over 3.7 million people are preppers.

The Prepper's Mindset

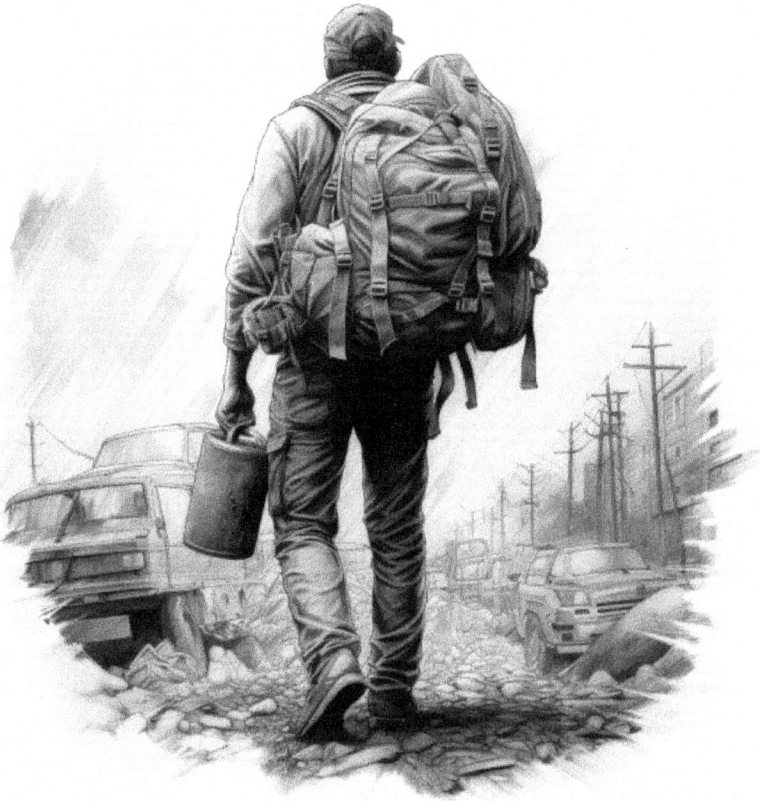

Tough living conditions do not defeat a prepper psychologically. As long as they are alive, preppers never give up hope or stop trying to survive, no matter the intensity of a disaster. The lack of doctors or conventional medicine doesn't freak them out about diseases. This is because they've already trained their body and mind to adapt to and cope with any situation.

Preppers don't grow desperate or panic when things get ugly. They are aware that losing hope of surviving kills faster than anything else. So, they always look for ways out, look for a cure, even when there seems to be none. This is why they prepare for when there are no doctors by learning about medicinal herbs and how to gain access in times of need.

Misconceptions About Prepping

Even prepping that doesn't incorporate herbs faces much ridicule, let alone trying to transition to plant-based medicine as a prepper. People may consider you to be

- paranoid

- crazy

- apocalyptic

- tight-fisted

- an underground bunker lone wolf

- a fearmonger

The majority of people who learn about prepping on TV tend to naturally form a negative opinion. Hence the negative connotations. People who condemn prepping probably never handled a life-threatening disaster personally. It's one thing to learn about disasters on TV from the comfort of your couch, but it's a different ballgame to experience them firsthand. When objectively examined, the misconceptions about prepping are unfounded.

Natural Medicine Connection With Prepping

All cultures have herbalists. Some common principles cherished by all herbalists include the following:

- A holistic approach to healthcare.

- A safe, least invasive, and most natural treatment.

- sustainable health management

- Appreciating the healing powers of nature.

- Eliminating the causes of sickness.

A Holistic Approach to Healthcare

Preppers also believe in these principles. The holistic approach to healthcare is to cure the entire body instead of certain parts or organs. This means using a single herb or collection of herbs to treat a range of illnesses or specific diseases while simultaneously boosting overall health. It's a fundamental principle of preparing to accomplish more with less.

The Safe, Least Invasive, and Most Natural Treatment

Herbalists strive for the safest, least invasive, and most natural treatment because they don't want side effects from their therapies. That's why they go for all-natural treatments. Prepping also emphasizes safety, ease, and harnessing the power of nature to solve problems. Using the safest approach is critical during a crisis because you don't want to create another problem while trying to solve one since resources will be limited.

Sustainable Health Management

If someone falls ill during a disaster, you don't want a solution that involves surgery since it'd be difficult to manage the wound and other post-surgery complications. Herbalists don't like invasive therapies like surgery, even under normal circumstances. Preppers, too, try to find and prepare the easiest health solutions.

Conventional medicine is expensive compared to the alternative. That makes it unsustainable for most people in the world today. We've seen how so many people went without healthcare during the Great Depression. Herbal medicine makes sustainable healthcare accessible to all since the knowledge is easy and cheap to acquire, and anybody can keep an herbal garden. Prepping asks you to look for sustainable solutions.

Appreciating the Healing Powers of Nature

Herbalists use as little conventional medicine as possible and only in the absence of a herbal alternative. I know a local herbalist who never goes to the hospital but manages his health, and his family's pretty well. He takes a certain plant powder in tea several times every three months or so to clean his gut.

This man never complains of gut issues despite doing very little exercise and leading a sedentary lifestyle. A friend of mine took his medicine twice, and his internal hemorrhoids disappeared for weeks. This man uses many other herbs for a range of diseases. According to him, these herbs fortify his body against diseases. Preppers strive to fortify themselves against future disasters and the problems they create.

Eliminating the Causes of Sickness

Herbalists usually want to find out the cause of a disease before trying to treat it. They want to eliminate the cause and symptom simultaneously. This is the best way to deal with an illness. When you eliminate the source and treat the symptom, you recover completely. For example, over-the-counter (OTC) ointments for hemorrhoids only manage the symptoms.

The herbalist I told you about treats hemorrhoids by purging the intestine of the harmful matter that clogs it. He instructs the patient to take the plant powder two or three times at the end of every month for about six consecutive months. Afterward, the patient can take it twice or so every three months. In addition to the plant powder, he prescribes a particular herbal ointment to shrink hemorrhoids and relieve pain. I came to realize that the powder prevents constipation by washing the gut clean of any sticky matter.

Our Ancestors Were Herbal Preppers

Before the advent of traditional medical practices, our ancestors grappled with illnesses and sought healing. The top 10 leading causes of death today are diseases, particularly heart disease. More people die from heart disease than ever before despite the great advances in medical practices (*WHO Reveals Leading Causes*, 2020). The leading causes of heart disease are obesity, lack of exercise, smoking, and poor diet. You can reduce the risks by leading a healthy lifestyle, such as by incorporating certain herbs into your diet (Mayo Clinic, n.d.).

Why didn't our ancestors die of heart disease in huge numbers like we do today, despite their less sophisticated healing practices? Herbs were their primary medicines, yet they were able to handle a wide range of diseases and injuries successfully. I'm not arguing that herbal medicine is better than conventional medicine. But it's clear that ancient people made better use of herbs, which was why they could overcome most diseases.

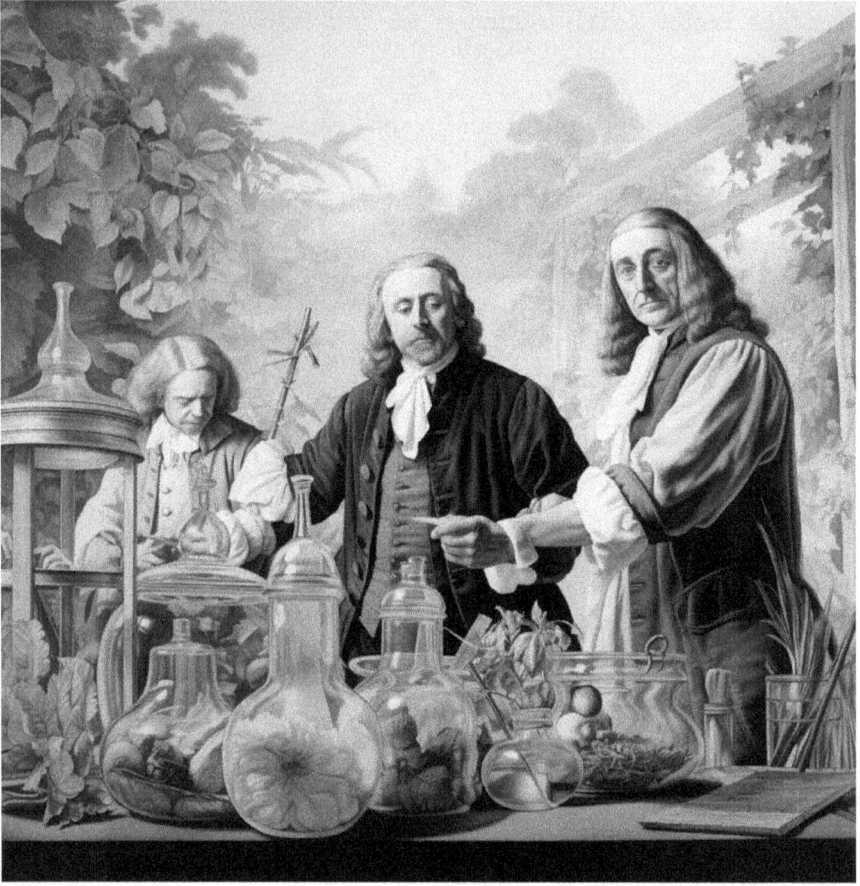

Some Herbs Are Going Extinct

If conventional medicine were to disappear all of a sudden, hundreds of millions would die within months, especially those who live on drugs. Yet, our ancestors lived for generations without conventional medicine. Did the herbs that preserve their health suddenly disappear or become impotent? We know that some 600 plant species have gone extinct in the last 250 years.

Thus, we have 600 fewer plants compared to the people who lived 250 years ago, which means fewer herbal remedies for us. I blame our overreliance on conventional medicine for this. Human activity, such as agriculture and climate change, caused the loss of most of these plants.

The Saint Helena olive is a flowering plant that disappeared in 2003. Scientists have warned that humans threaten the existence of hundreds of thousands of plant species today (Briggs, 2019).

Prepping Can Slow Down Plant Extinction

Preppers can help preserve some endangered plants. Prepping and naturopathy share the same principle. Both aim to make an individual self-reliant health-wise. However, prepping goes a lot further by making the individual completely independent in terms of food, water, shelter, clothing, and health. Naturopathy focuses on health only and promotes a healthy lifestyle and the use of herbs for healing (Better Health Channel, 2012).

Herbal Prepping for Every Situation

Let's see a few examples where herbal medicine know-how can be critical to survival.

When You Travel

Mishandling any crisis has the potential to be life-threatening, cause enduring health issues, or severely disrupt one's life, contingent upon its timing and location. A health situation can arise after your car breaks down in the middle of nowhere or while hiking, camping, hunting, or traveling. Maybe no one will show up for days or even weeks. If you don't presently have the right pill bottle or are unable to positively identify plant medicine in nature that can help control the situation, you may face a life-threatening danger.

During a Severe Crisis

The above examples, while life-threatening, are mild as they are easier to find help with than other emergencies. But these aren't the crises I want to help you prepare for. My focus is on emergencies you can't easily find help with. I classify such crises as *severe* because their effects are far-reaching and can seriously disrupt or cut access to healthcare.

During a severe crisis, the grid or one of its critical components can collapse or become overloaded. Our healthcare buckled under the 2020 pandemic, as did that of many other countries. It was terrible, and you must prepare for a repeat of that or something worse. Take steps to reduce and eventually eliminate your dependence on the healthcare system or big pharma.

In Your Homestead

Sicknesses can occur while you are at home and without enough money for treatment. Or it may happen in your homestead, and you can't transport the victim to a hospital immediately. For example, malaria and typhoid fever are highly deadly combinations that occur at the same time and need treatment right away. If you don't maintain any medical preps or an herbal garden for a range of diseases, you may soon mourn a loved one.

Prepping With Conventional Medicine

You can choose to stock up on pharmaceutical drugs for malaria, flu, ulcers, etc. It's possible to stockpile enough for several months or years. However, you'll still likely succumb to diseases and injuries in an emergency. The reason is that conventional medicine has several downsides that make it unreliable for long-term health crises. Some downsides include the following:

- an unreliable source

- a vulnerable supply chain

- a limited shelf life

- Treatment isn't holistic

- requires in-depth knowledge

- high chances of side effects

- often limited quantity

An Unreliable Source

Your normal medicines originate from an unreliable source. The need for a manufacturing facility and a trained workforce makes it difficult to produce these medicines. Depending on the intensity of the crisis, pharmaceutical companies and skilled labor may not be available. For example, after Russian air and missile strikes targeted energy facilities in some Ukrainian cities, manufacturing industries ground to a halt, crippling the pharmaceutical industry.

Supply Chain Issues and Shelf Life

But even if some drug manufacturers operated during a huge crisis, distribution would be difficult or impossible. Big Pharma's reliance on long supply chains opens it to sudden disruptions and closures. Additionally, you may easily end up with a bunch of expired pills or syrups in your bug-out bag or medical pantry. This happens as a result of the limited shelf life of most pharmaceuticals.

Non-Holistic Treatment and Other Problems

Conventional medicines usually treat a specific disease only, making them less holistic than plant-based remedies. A holistic approach to healing is one of the main differences between natural and man-made therapies.

Conventional drugs are also more likely to have side effects. Their main ingredients are often highly concentrated and do not work with the support of other compounds. They are isolated compounds and most require in-depth knowledge to be used correctly. One must train as a pharmacist, medical doctor, or other related field to prescribe or administer conventional medicines. That isn't the case with herbal remedies. Anyone can become a world-class herbalist with less than a year of training and practice.

Pharmaceuticals are less available than their green counterparts. In an emergency, they are likely to disappear or become very expensive. Additionally, anyone can cultivate herbs in large quantities. Plant-based medicine has the exact opposite of all the downsides bullet-pointed above. A single plant or group of plants can usually treat or help manage a range of diseases, which lets you do more with less and ultimately conserve space in your stockpile.

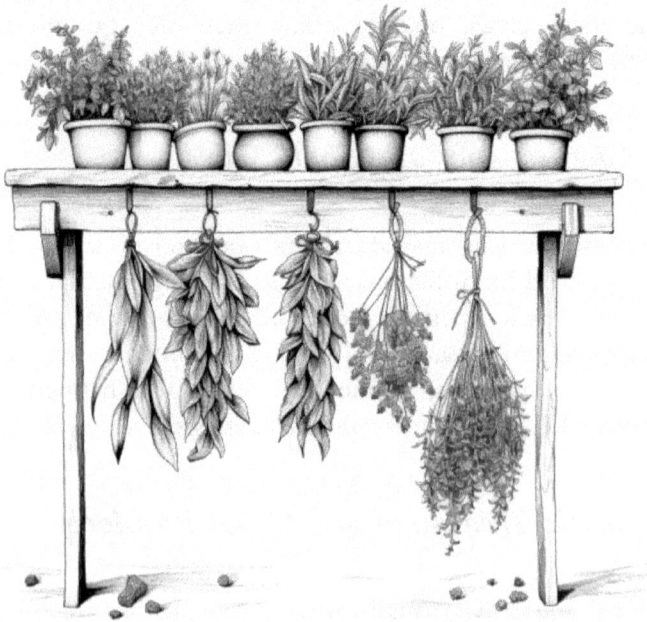

Independent Wellness

Amid a crisis, relying solely on conventional drugs can limit your ability to fully manage your health due to several inherent drawbacks. Supplementing with plant-based remedies can easily give you this control, provided you won't mind a little exercise in a garden or bush and some reading. It's a great idea to start incorporating plant medicine into your health and diet regimen now to lessen the challenges of a potential future switch.

Collaborate with a qualified doctor when incorporating herbs into your life, especially if you have an underlying health condition or are currently receiving treatment (including before and after surgery). Herbs can interfere with certain drugs or healing processes, like blood clotting. This is why your doctor must approve any plant-based remedies you use.

Why Embrace Plant-Based Therapies

Actively testing natural health solutions will reveal how your system reacts to different herbs. Plants that cause serious allergies or illnesses can be substituted, transformed, or doses calibrated to a safer threshold. The goal is to figure out what works best for you and how much to take so you know exactly what to include in your preps and what to do in a crisis. It'd be wonderful if we fully transitioned to plant-based medicine. Naturopathy provides significant advantages before, during, and after a crisis. Here are a few of its benefits:

- Plants are natural.

- they are sustainable

- they are easy to produce

- they can be 100% organic

- they save you money

- some are delicious (teas)

- they are nutritious

- environmentally friendly

- easy to prepare

- have long shelf lives

- rarely produce side effects

- cure multiple diseases

- enhance overall health

- relatively easy to learn

- many are highly effective (*cabbage juice vs. antacids* for ulcers)

Conclusion

Acquiring the knowledge of growing and using plants for medicine and nutrition is a critical skill for every prepper. Your preparation isn't complete without this crucial tool in your tool belt. If you research thoroughly online, you'll discover many instances where disaster victims relied on plants for medicine and even food. They couldn't have effectively used any plants whose medicinal uses were unknown to them. Your knowledge of growing and using herbs is way more important than your herbal stockpiles. It's secure from thieves and damage, and it weighs less than a feather.

Therefore, ignore any stereotypes against prepping or herbal medicine. Study, practice, and stockpile herbs. It's a finite process with lifelong rewards. In chapter two, I'll teach you how to empower wellness with plants. You'll learn plenty about natural remedies and discover the medical uses of many plants. Keep reading!

Chapter 2:

Herbal Medicine—Tracing Its Path

Through History and

Contemporary Times

To keep the body in good health is a duty, otherwise we shall not be able to keep our mind strong and clear. –Buddha

The origin of herbal medicine traces back to the earliest humans, who also battled diseases and injuries as we do today. Much of the modern world's herbal knowledge came from our ancestors, who lived hundreds or thousands of years ago. Developing nations use herbs the most and without credible research, meaning the herbs aren't scientifically cross-examined. Let's take a brief look at the journey of herbal medicine from the earliest generations to the 21st century.

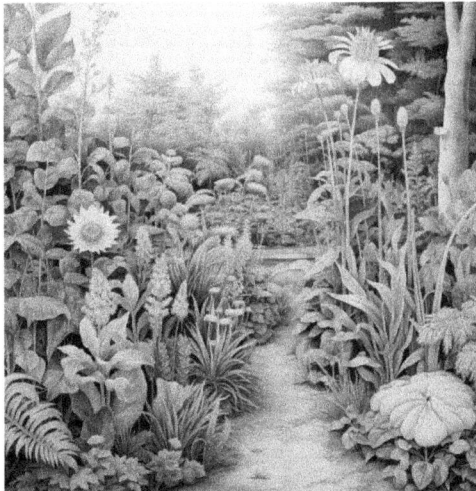

How Humans Started Using Herbal Medicine

Medicine predates mankind, dating back to the existence of plants that precede our species. Human survival across diverse environments has spurred an eternal quest for nature's remedies and wellness. Numerous factors, both internal and external, pose challenges to human health. Consequently, there's an enduring pursuit to comprehend the human body, its surroundings, and any elements that could endanger or enhance life.

The human discovery of plant medicine was purely accidental. It was by eating raw and cooked plants, including non-edible ones, that people found some plants had a desired effect on their body, such as alleviating pain, boosting energy, or ending illnesses. Hence, all early discoveries came through real-life experience (Petrovska, 2012).

The lack of historical records indicates a conspicuous absence of details regarding the causes and symptoms of a disease, let alone its treatment, during the early phases of herbal medicine usage. *Experience* was the basis for all discoveries, as opposed to our accurate scientific experiments today. Herbalism was the only form of therapy until the 16th century.

Preserving and Expanding Herbalism

People passed on knowledge of plant medicine from generation to generation by word of mouth. This was because the first users of herbal medicine did not document their discoveries—perhaps due to limited herbal knowledge, illiteracy, and documentation resources. However, humans eventually started keeping records of the names of certain plants and their medicinal uses in a bid to preserve a growing knowledge bank.

We aren't the only generation that studies the human body and environment for health reasons. People of all eras did that albeit in different ways. Archeologists, scientists, and historians have discovered monuments, documents, and remains of plant medicines, some dating as far back as 60,000 years ago.

Just like we try to study herbal medical history today, so did other generations. Usually, every generation outshines the previous one's understanding of medicinal herbs as it combines previous knowledge with present discoveries. The incremental additions to previous knowledge led to our modern pharmaceutical drugs.

Documentation of Herbal Medicine Know-How

Our only scientific evidence for the first herbal medical documentation is the Sumerian clay slabs from Nagpur dated 5000 years ago. The documents show how to prepare certain herbal remedies using 12 recipes concocted from over 250 plants, including alkaloids like mandrake, poppy, and henbane among others. Documentation might have started earlier, but there's no sufficient evidence in that regard.

In 2500 BC, the Chinese emperor, Shen Nung, wrote an herbal medicine book titled *Pen T'Sao*—Chinese for "Roots and Grass"—describing 365 drugs from plants, some of which are still used in China today. Some of the plants featured in this book are ephedra, rhei rhizoma, cinnamon bark, camphor, jimson weed, theae folium, and ginseng. Information on herbal medicine can also be found in the Indian holy book, the Vedas, which mentions plants like pepper, nutmeg, clove, and more.

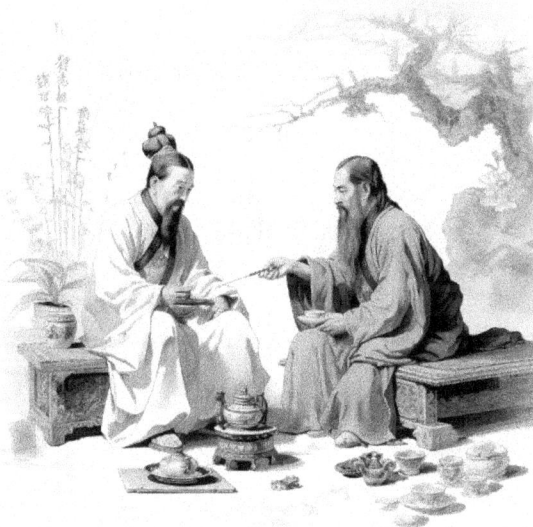

The Ebers Papyrus contains over 800 prescriptions derived from 700 plant species and features plants like garlic, juniper, willow, and others. Even the Bible and Talmud mention using plants for rituals that go with certain therapies.

Herbalism Becomes More Sophisticated

Written work on plant medicine later got more sophisticated as people like Theophrastus began classifying herbal plants according to a set of criteria. His books "De Historia Plantarum" and "De Causis Plantarium" laid the foundation for botanical science. He advocated for a gradual adaptation to traditional herbal remedies by advising individuals to incrementally increase their doses, allowing their systems to acclimate.

A time came when pharmacognosists started traveling long distances to study the herbs of other traditions. Dioscorides was the most prominent writer who combined herbs from different traditions in his writings. That earned him the title of the father of pharmacognosy—the branch of knowledge concerned with medicinal drugs obtained from plants or other natural sources. He was a military physician for the Roman army. In 77 AD, he wrote the book "De Materia Medica" It was widely translated and served as the primary medical book for all civilizations back then until the late Middle Ages and the Renaissance.

Herbalism Incorporates Minerals and Animals

Dioscorides described 944 drugs, 657 of which were plant-based. Drugs derived from animal and mineral sources accounted for the remaining substances. Dioscorides' work provides a good glimpse of when non-plant medicine started to be used. Dioscorides' contribution to pharmacognosy is unparalleled. He excelled at consolidating therapies from different traditions, including non-plant medicines, and provided detailed information on each herb, such as locality, outward appearance, preparation, harvesting, and so on.

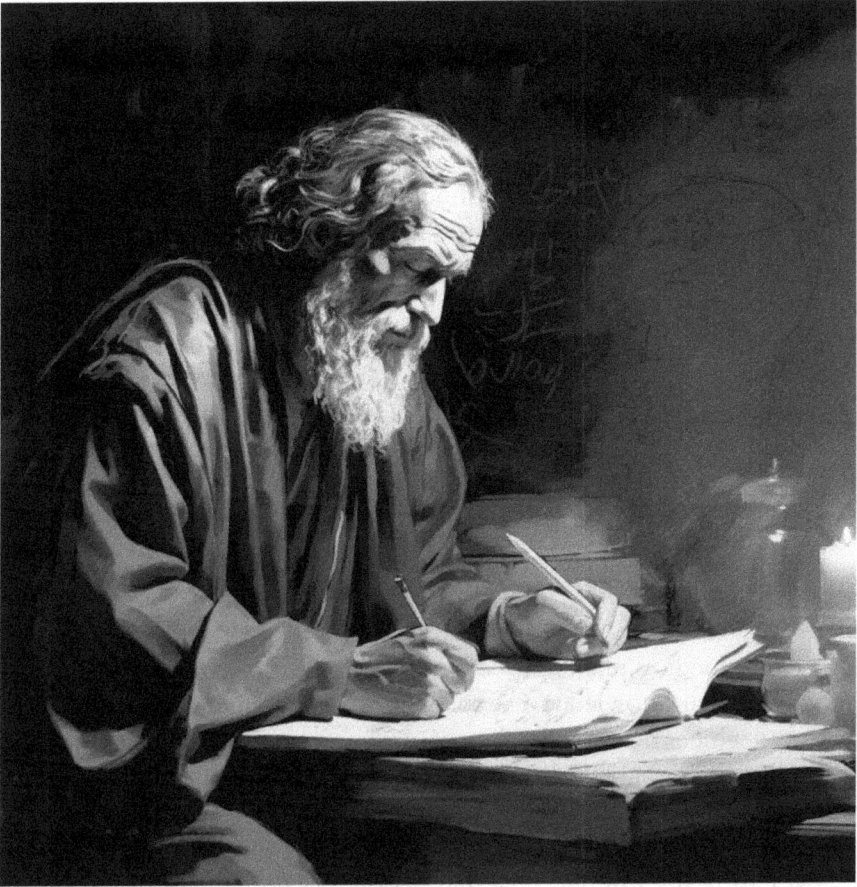

So, physicians went on writing books on pharmacognosy. Some introduced a more advanced order to their work, such as the Roman physician Galen (131 AD–200), who was the first to group herbs by similarity in action. This grouping is what we refer to as *parallel drugs* today. His aim was to make it easier for people to find alternative plants.

False Believes on Herbal Medicines

Dioscorides made certain medical claims that turned out to be wrong but were widely believed by many generations. He said *Camomile* or *Chamaemelon* had abortive actions, but modern scientific research has debunked this claim. Such cases are the reason some people don't have confidence in herbal medicine while others go as far as condemning herbalism. I'll address this issue briefly later.

The Roman Empire and other pagan-based traditions tended to attribute sickness to spiritual problems and divine punishment. Around 400 BC, some pharmacognosists, like Hippocrates, initiated a critical reevaluation of the notion of attributing illnesses to supernatural causes. Hippocrates stood firmly for the argument that diseases originated from the body and proposed separating religion from medicine. As a result of challenging official beliefs, Hippocrates' efforts to separate religion from medicine were met with lifetime imprisonment (Roots of Western Herbalism, 2019).

Herbal Medical Knowledge Converges in Europe

Throughout the Middle Ages, Europe's medical knowledge flourished under Arab influence, predominantly through pivotal texts discussing over 1,000 medical plants. As Marco Polo toured the world, he amassed herbal medical knowledge from Persia, India, China, and other Asian cultures, which he took back to Europe. The Europeans continued accumulating herbal insights from all over the world, including America after it was discovered.

It was during the Middle Ages that people began to cultivate medicinal herbs and dedicate official institutions to consolidating, maintaining, administering, and teaching herbal medicine. Monasteries were pivotal hubs for herbalism and therapeutic practices, focusing on 16 primary plants, including tansy, sage, savory, mint, Greek seed, and several others. Medical schools like Salerno would later be established for growing herbs on state-owned lands and training herbalists.

In the 15th century, some physicians started advocating the chemical production of drugs from plant, animal, and mineral sources. By the 18th century, the demand for chemically prepared drugs was particularly huge. These compound drugs were more expensive as they contained plant, animal, and mineral ingredients. By the late 19th and early 20th centuries, chemical drugs threatened to take over the therapeutic market (Petrovska, 2012).

A Snapshot of Herbalism in America

Advanced herbal knowledge first reached Europe before America. America's herbal know-how came largely from the Europeans, who in turn got theirs mainly from the Arabs. The indigenous peoples of America had been using herbal medicine for centuries before the arrival of Christopher Columbus. Europe copied their healing knowledge, and later introduced it to America.

Some enslaved Africans brought their traditional herbal knowledge, which they shared with the locals until it spread over wide areas. Cottage herbalists and midwives also contributed to the development of America's herbalism, which became very advanced by the 19th century.

Herbalist's Irreversible Decline

It was during the 19th century that American physicians started making a significant shift from plant-only medicines to what they called "heroic medicines." "Heroic" because these medicines had faster and more powerful effects, thanks to the concentrated compounds that specifically targeted diseases. In other words, treatment becomes non-holistic. These new cures came from plants and mineral sources, including toxic substances like mercury and arsenic. Those were the conventional physicians, and they fully adopted analytical chemistry as a barrier every medicine must go through to be accepted (*18th Century Book*, n.d.).

In other words, every herb must pass through the laboratory, regardless of its previous effectiveness. However, some unconventional physicians, like physio-medicalists and eclectics opposed this new condition, opting for innovative solutions that are plant-based and less invasive. Fierce competition emerged between the proponents and critics of plant-only medicines. They fought for patients, reputation, and prominence until the 1930s, when new official laws tilted the balance against unconventional physicians.

From 1910 to 1935, universities had to drop all unconventional medical courses or risk losing accreditation. This was the last nail in the coffin for the official support of herbalism. Chemically produced drugs officially took over to this very day. The justification for this government-backed move against herbalism was unscientific in light of today's realities as we'll find out soon.

Herbalism Today

Did herbalism disappear in America after the US government implicitly withdrew support for herbal medicine and literally battered it into a comma in the 1930s? How far has herbalism gone today in America and around the world? How about claims that herbal medicine is better (not necessarily more effective) than pharmaceutical drugs?" "What about people who want big pharma to permanently stifle herbal medicine? We'll briefly answer these questions to help you get the most out of herbs as a prepper.

Herbalism in 21st-century America

The government stopped short of outlawing herbalism in America for fear of the public outcry that would inevitably follow and for a lack of credible scientific justification. At least one motive of the conventional physicians who pushed for ending government support for herbalism was to monopolize medicinal knowledge. The healthcare industry wasn't so lucrative during the era of herbalism. Attempts to restrict herbal knowledge date back to the 15th century when Nicholas Culpeper angered many physicians with his mission to make medical knowledge freely available to all.

Nicholas Culpeper was an English astrologer, herbalist, physician, botanist, and apothecary (pharmacist). He was a threat to the businesses of herbalists who wanted to monopolize medical knowledge. They tried stopping him without success but managed to get him tried twice for witchcraft, which nearly got him barred from practice. It's obvious that profit-driven conventional physicians managed to monopolize medicinal knowledge when they undermined public confidence in the efficacy of herbal medicines back in the 30s and persuaded the government to withdraw support for herbalism.

But herbalism made a comeback during the 60s and 70s, with its popularity continuing to soar since then. It's even made inroads into conventional medicine. The integrative or functional medicine movement is playing a critical role in driving public consciousness and acceptance of herbalism. This movement advocates for integrating herbalism and conventional medicine.

Herbalism Around the World

Eighty-eight percent of some African and Asian countries use herbals as their primary medicine. Most governments didn't support conventional medicine over unconventional medicine like the American and European governments did in the early 20th century. Therefore, herbal medicine continues to be a highly valued commodity for healthcare and wellness in many countries. Herbal cure varies among different cultures due to factors influencing herbalism, such as geographic location, traditional beliefs and theories, evolution, and so on (*Catalysing Ancient Wisdom*, 2023).

I expect the use of herbals in developed nations to increase to the point òf competing favorably with conventional medicine, as we see in many countries today. This is because sickness is widespread at a time of difficult financial situations for most humans and the worsening inability of pharmaceutical drugs to deal with the illnesses plaguing the world. A holistic approach to health and wellness, in addition to conventional medicine, offers the best chance against chronic diseases.

Is It True That Herbals Are Largely Ineffective?

This is one of the most important questions that shapes decisions about harnessing nature's protective and healing powers. We've briefly studied herbs from a historical perspective. It's time to quickly go over some scientific and logical facts about herbs. I don't want us to *assume* that herbs are effective. That's because a significant number of people are unsure about using herbs.

As such, a solid understanding of the effectiveness of herbal medicines is necessary to use them confidently. Confidence is critical to balancing your mind and body for effective treatment and prevention. Here are some reasons to get or keep you on the positive side of herbals:

- availability of scientific proofs

- big pharma raw materials

- formal professional courses

- recommended by doctors and pharmacists

- widespread anecdotal evidence

Availability of Scientific Findings

The sudden popularity of herbs has prompted scientists to run experiments to confirm or refute their efficacy. As a result, thousands of studies have been conducted on plants for scientific proof of their medical benefits. The majority of these studies were able to silence critics of herbal therapies. Here are a few examples among thousands:

- Tabassum and Ahmad (2011) clinically proved that the leaf extracts of the Annona muricata tree lower elevated blood pressure.

- The gum Arabic tree, prickly chaff flower, acosmium, and several other plants clinically demonstrated strong anti-diabetes properties (Kooti et al., 2016).

- Cabbage juice can cure ulcers caused by the notorious H. Pylori bacteria (Fahey et al., 2015).

Big Pharma Raw Materials

Chemical analysis was invented in the late 18th century and saw several improvements starting in the early 19th century (*Analytical Chemistry*, 2018). Since then, chemists have used the method to extract and purify certain plant ingredients for their pharmaceuticals. Many conventional drugs still widely use plants as raw materials today. In fact, a fourth of Big Pharma's raw materials come from plants (Herbal Medicine Information, n.d.).

Formal Professional Courses

Universities and colleges around the world continue to introduce herbal medicine courses as independent disciplines or supplementary courses to traditional medical fields. At least nine Western universities and colleges offer herbal medicine courses (9 Institutions Offering, n.d.). The goal is to train herbal medical professionals who can combine herbs and conventional drugs in their therapies.

Recommended by Doctors and Pharmacists

Some doctors and pharmacists have received training in herbal medicine and are recommending some alternative treatments to patients. As a result, they create treatment plans that combine herbs, lifestyle adjustments, and conventional medicine for a range of health conditions.

Widespread Anecdotal Evidence

The study I mentioned at the beginning of this chapter showed that about 68% of respondents (students) favored incorporating herbs into conventional medical services. Most of the respondents said they've used herbs to treat malaria, typhoid, and other diseases (Nworu et al., 2015).

One-third of Americans have used herbs for treatment in the past few decades. The most visible popularity of herbs is in the supplement industry. Amazon is full of supplement products for a range of health benefits, and people buy millions of packages every year. Entire industries are built around herbalism due to its broad scope.

Can Herbs Substitute for Pharmaceuticals?

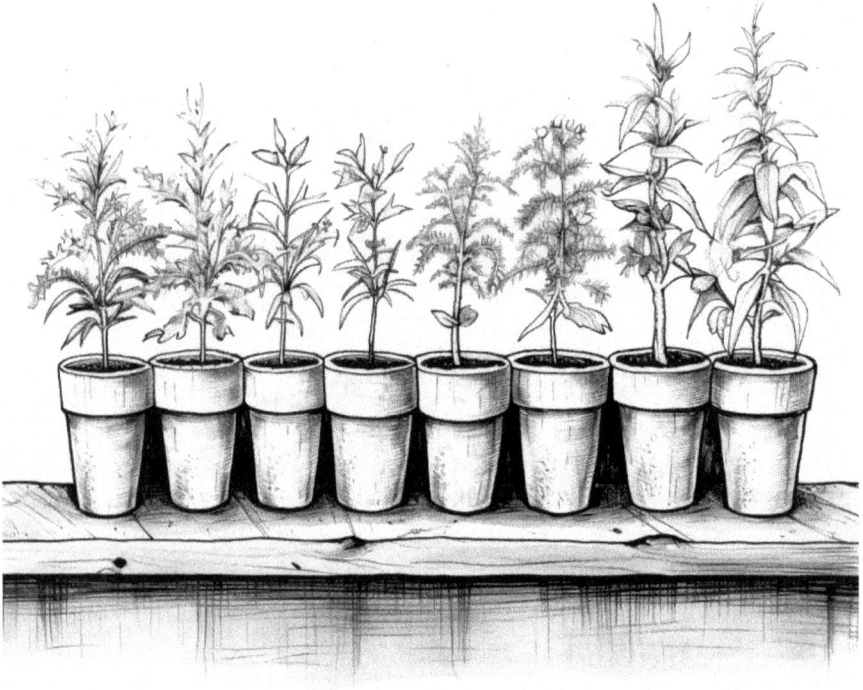

Yes, because some people have done it successfully. Our ancestors survived without pharmaceutical drugs and lived healthy lives. In the last chapter of this book, I'll explain how to transition from conventional to herbal medicines for those who want to try. However, obtaining your doctor's consent is essential. The goal is to significantly improve overall health with lifestyle and dietary changes that include herbs. We'll cover many herbs in this book, including the critical ones.

Many people are taking herbs as supplements, especially those with cancer, stroke, arthritis, obesity, respiratory illnesses, and other chronic diseases. Supplements are just fancy forms of medicinal herbs. 12% of Americans used herbs in the late 90s. The US sold herbal products worth over $5.3 billion in 2012. In 2013, this figure increased by 8%. Most people said they used herbs to independently manage their health problems, improve general wellness, and live longer. That means, in a way, many supplement users think like herbal preppers (Rashrash, 2017).

It's important to know certain facts in order to ground your understanding in knowledge. However, the fact that herbal medicine has many critics motivates me to provide a waterproof backup for my conclusions. I'd rather present facts that lead to a logical conclusion than expect you to take my word for it as a fellow prepper or fan. Here are some points to ponder regarding whether our ancestors relied primarily on herbs for healthcare.

They Had Reasons to Seek Cure

Our ancestors must have been forced to seek cures in order to survive due to several main reasons.

- **Diseases**: We have scientific, historical, and logical proof that diseases, pains, and injuries existed long before analytical chemistry. In case you forgot, analytical chemistry is the branch of chemistry that gave rise to the pharmaceutical drugs and chemical products we have today. Scientists have documented over 1000 historical diseases our ancestors likely grappled with. They also had pathogens, viruses, bacteria, mosquitoes, tsetse flies, and other disease-causing organisms.

- **Wounds**: Since ancient times, humans have been engaged in the ongoing struggle of warfare. That means soldiers and even civilians suffered mild and severe wounds like cuts and stabs, which would get infected if not treated. Accidents did happen in pre-modern generations. They also fell from trees and cliffs, into pits and ditches, from horseback and chariots, and so on. Some victims fractured or broke a bone, twisted a joint, or bumped a muscle. Some wounds required treatment.

- **Poisons**: Earlier generations have had to deal with poisons and poisonous substances—both natural and man-made. There were cases of food and water contamination, leading to instances where individuals might have unknowingly consumed toxic plants or substances. They had snakes, dangerous insects, and weapons fortified with poison.

If primitive generations could successfully cope with the above issues by using herbs, it means we can do it too. The biggest challenge is finding the right herbs, which this book aims to teach you, in addition to discussing a large number of medicinal herbs you can grow or obtain in America. As a prepper, you are getting ready to handle these issues if they arise during an emergency, especially a prolonged crisis.

They Didn't Have Advanced Laboratories

It was only after the invention of analytical chemistry that humans began building advanced laboratories for studying diseases and medicines at the microscopic level. Our ancestors didn't have these laboratories, which means they couldn't study diseases and medicines in depth. They had doctors, nurses, and primitive laboratories which eventually evolved into our modern research facilities. So, since they didn't have advanced clinical facilities like us, they had to come up with other ways of discovering medicines and treating diseases and injuries. We'll briefly study their methods in the next section.

Herbs Are Medically Effective

Primitive doctors were certain to stumble over effective herbal cures while dealing with diseases and injuries. We already understood that herbs are medicinally effective based on scientific research and other facts. The chances of herbal doctors and researchers discovering effective treatments for diseases and injuries must've been high, considering their proximity to a variety of plants, some of which are extinct today. Once herbal doctors and researchers discover a cure, they are unlikely to forget it.

Archeological Findings on Herbs

Over the years, archeologists have recovered remains of herbal medicine dating as far back as 60,000 years ago (McKenna, 2010). Papyrus writings of ancient Chinese and Egyptian societies showed the medicinal uses of certain plants as early as 3000 BC. Other archeological findings suggest that people used herbs in Scotland as early as the Bronze Age. These are sufficient proofs that ancient people studied and used herbs for medicine.

Our Forefathers Were Herbal Preppers

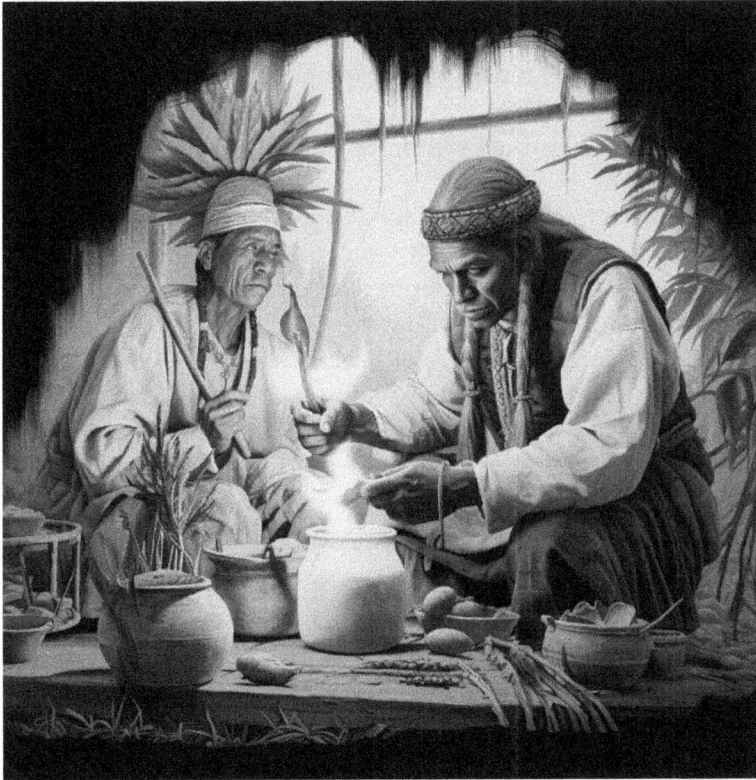

Our forefathers just didn't nickname it *herbal prepping*. Drawn from their teachings and historical documentation, it seems the core of natural medicine for them was to empower everyone as an herbal prepper capable of self-care. Naturopathic doctors (NDs) serve as both healers and educators, emphasizing that lifelong wellness demands personal knowledge of naturopathy. Our immune system, our frontline defense, requires continual maintenance like any other bodily system. Herbalism taps into nature's power, utilizing plants, exercises, and the environment to maintain and enhance our immune system, preventing and curing illnesses.

The Philosophy and Principles of Herbal Medicine

The approach of naturopathy to treatment is to fix the body as a whole rather than in parts. Naturopathy doesn't present two or more treatment options for a disease. There's only one way to treat the disease, and that is to eliminate the cause and symptom simultaneously.

On the other hand, conventional medicine focuses on the symptom and the affected part. For example, if someone has external hemorrhoids, conventional therapy recommends several options for dealing with them. One option is to buy OTC medication that relieves pain and shrinks the hemorrhoids. Another option is surgery. The third option can be rubber-band ligation that removes the hemorrhoids. A fourth option is an injection that shrinks the hemorrhoids. In most cases, all these would be temporary fixes. Doctors would also advise you on lifestyle and diet changes, but that won't be a major side of the treatment. All the treatment options use pharmaceutical drugs, which have their disadvantages, as seen earlier.

The Concept of Naturopathy

Naturopathy recommends herbs instead of an OTC or pharmaceutical drug to deal with the symptoms and causes. It prioritizes herbs, lifestyle and diet changes, and things you should always or often do to pre-empt it or at least significantly reduce the chances. Herbs target the symptom, cause, and strength of organs as a bonus. Naturopathy doesn't want treatment to taste, smell, or feel like treatment. That eliminates or minimizes any inconvenience. Therapy that comes with inconvenience is not sustainable. You want it to end as soon as possible to spare you those pills and hospital trips.

In summary, the moment you get sick, naturopathy says there's a problem with your lifestyle and/or what you *consume* or *don't* consume. For example, hemorrhoids would mean you do little physical activity, eat a lot of processed food, take little water, or lack some *delicious* herbs that prevent constipation among many other benefits. You may be violating one or more of these natural rules of optimal and enduring health.

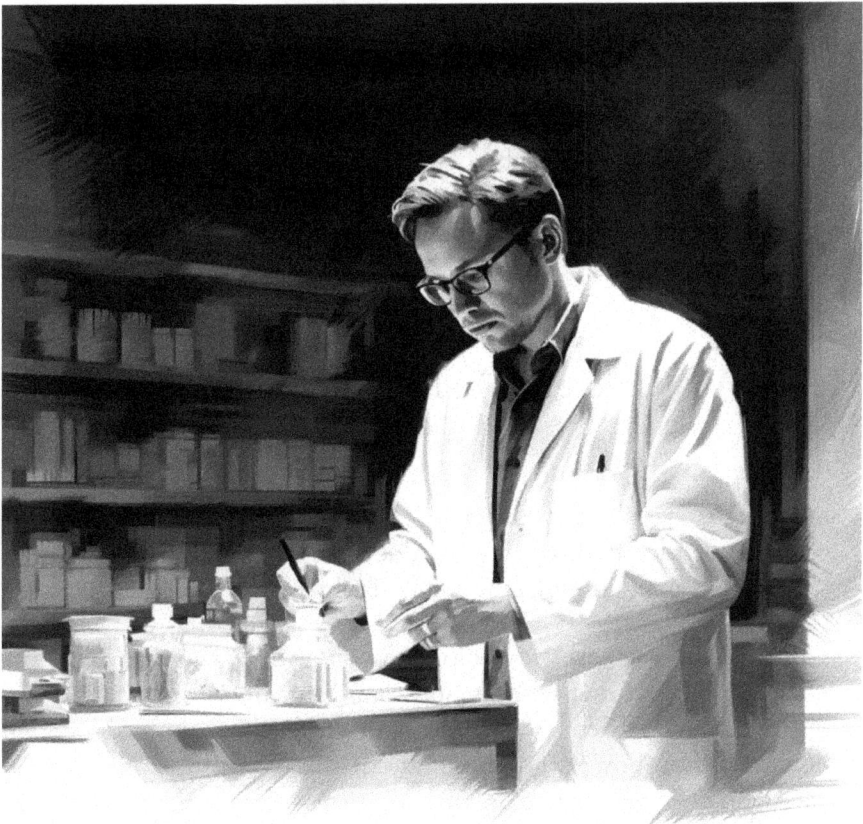

Herbals Needn't Taste, Smell, or Feel Bad

Note that herbs are delicious or can be made so. I'll teach you some tricks to make teas, juices, and soups out of herbs. Herbs are cheap enough to be considered free. In sharp contrast, most pharmaceuticals smell like chemicals and taste weird, and nothing you do would change that. They are also relatively expensive, and many are unaffordable for the average dude. On the other hand, *all* herbal medicines can be transformed into delicious tea, juice, or soup, and they are within reach of even the poorest people on the planet.

So here's the deal, folks: it's important to regularly incorporate protective, preventive, and health-boosting herbs into your diet in a delightful, flavorful way. You can get creative about transforming those herbs or simply take them in your coffee, food, or beverage. It won't even remotely feel like taking medicine. I recommend growing a garden to have a large variety of fresh and dry herbs around. The right collection of herbs will protect your health better than any supplement or drug you can ever find. Couple this with an active lifestyle, and your chances of sickness decrease radically. As a prepper, you can stockpile as much as you want from a garden.

Herbal Vs. Conventional Medicine for Preppers

- Herbs won't contain any chemicals if grown organically. Conventional drugs are products of chemical processes and usually contain minerals, some of which aren't safe.

- You can use herbs for as long as you want or even make them a part of your diet without spending a fortune. All you need is a well-kept garden, some foraging, or a reliable supply source. I'll teach you how to go about any of these. On the contrary, you won't *optionally* use pharmaceuticals for long—except for supplements, which usually contain undeclared substances and can cost a lot, especially family plans.

- Herbs are delightful to take, especially if you work on the form, taste, and scent. But most drugs must be gulped down your throat, sometimes with an effort. Ever heard of *pill phagophobia*? It refers to the fear of swallowing pills. Many people have it, and it's a hot keyword in Google searches. People are mostly looking for ways to deal with it.

- Drugs target specific illnesses and don't usually offer bonus health benefits—side effects are more likely. Herbs are holistic in medical action. You get vitamins, antioxidants, calories, etc., alongside the compounds that attack your disease. This is why herbalists say herbs treat the entire system.

- Herbs give you total control, while pharmaceutical drugs can only be purchased or received on humanitarian grounds. A 32-square-foot herbal garden is sufficient for a family of 5. You decide which, when, and how much herbs to use in your foods and beverages.

- You can forage for herbs if your garden is too far or inaccessible. Thankfully, most herbs grow in the wild, in bushes, and in uncultivated lands. You just need to be able to recognize and use them correctly. Later on, my plan is to provide you with the theoretical knowledge for foraging herbs.

Potential Risks With Herbs

An improper approach to herbalism can be deadly. This was the case of 37-year-old Seema Pravin Haribhai, who decided to try herbal remedies for arthritis. Her sickness was becoming increasingly disabling despite strict conventional therapy. Haribhai lost confidence in her conventional medication and wanted to transition to herbs. The Ayurveda practitioner she consulted recommended certain herbal remedies that damaged Haribhai's liver after she took it for several days.

Haribhai violated three rules for transitioning from conventional to herbal remedies, which contributed to her demise. She did not seek professional medical advice; she didn't research the content and side effects of her herbals; and she started with full doses. Impurities and harmful compounds aren't the only risks with plant medicine. Herbals that are good for one person can be dangerous for another. That's why you must follow the right procedure when incorporating herbs (Kirk, 2022).

Conclusion

It's clear now that herbs are medically effective and have been the primary medicine for thousands of years. All their discoveries were based on experience. Our ancestors managed to transfer medicinal knowledge by word of mouth or documentation to subsequent generations, some of whom have survived right up to the 21st century. We have more advanced and less risky procedures today. However dire the situation, people can resort to "experience" as a successful means of finding a cure. This would mean testing the herbs for effectiveness—in small, non-lethal doses or consuming them as food and taking note of any extraordinary health improvements as a result.

I don't wish for it or intend to spread fear, but there might come a time when Western civilization faces a complete collapse, perhaps due to a global conflict like a potential World War III. Renowned historian Arnold J. Toynbee cautioned about this very scenario. Governments could crumble, leading to a breakdown in nationwide law and order. In such a situation, hospitals or laboratories for testing the effectiveness of medicinal herbs might cease to exist. Whether we're individuals who prepare for emergencies or simply intrigued by the concept of preparedness, we strive to prepare ourselves for a future where these institutions might not exist. If prehistoric societies managed, there's no reason we shouldn't be capable of doing the same.

Chapter 3:

Unveiling Nature's Pharmacy—A

Detailed Herbal Compendium

Nature itself is the best physician. –Hippocrates

Here's where you will learn about many herbs in order to know how to obtain and use them. I've described no fewer than 90 herbs with information on their medicinal uses, side effects, native habitat, the parts to harvest or use, recommended doses, preparations, and how to consume them. Each herb has references for you to verify any information before using the herb. I took great caution to ensure these texts are factual, but don't consider anything here as professional medical advice.

Consult a healthcare professional before taking any of these herbs, especially if you are pregnant, nursing, or on medications. Herbs can be as powerful as conventional medicines, which means they can pose life-threatening risks if misused. Unless you are allergic to a plant, taking medication it interferes with, or consuming excess amounts, side effects are rare.

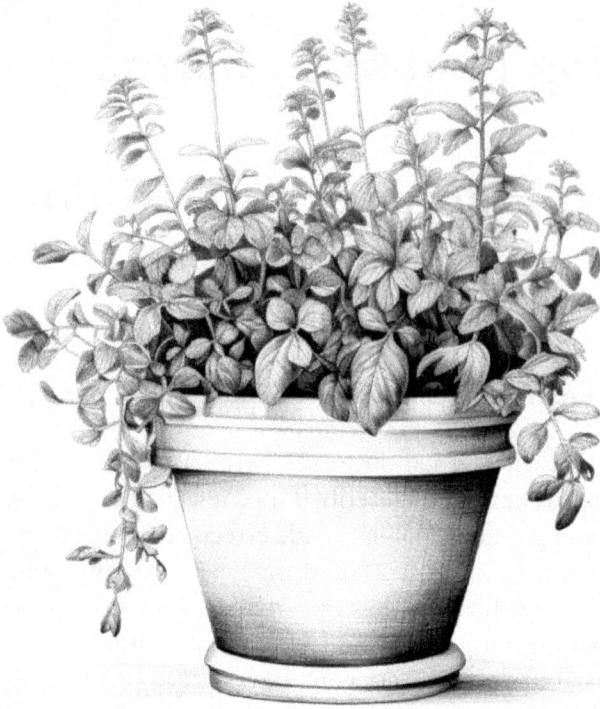

Allspice

- **Healing applications**: colds, nasal congestion, menstrual cramps, headache, indigestion, fatigue, menopause, cancer, bacterial and fungal infections, weight loss, bloating, and blood sugar

- **Side effects**: Potential adverse reactions include hives, swelling of the lips or tongue, shortness of breath, wheezing, vomiting, and diarrhea.

- **Native habitat**: It originated in the Caribbean, Central America, and South America and can be cultivated in Florida, Texas, California, Hawaii, Louisiana, Georgia, South Carolina, Alabama,

Mississippi, Arizona, Puerto Rico, the U.S. Virgin Islands, and others.

- **Part(s) used**: Pick the berries from the plant's flower and sundry them to a brown color.

- **Preparation**: You can grind it to powder or use the berries whole. Add this as an ingredient in your meals, or consume it alone.

- **Recommended dosage**: It's a spice without any recommended dosage. Use it appropriately in your recipes.

- **Application methods**: The powder adds a peppery flavor and enhances the taste of stews, poultry, meats, and vegetables. You can also use the powder for baking (Jones & Lang, 2021b).

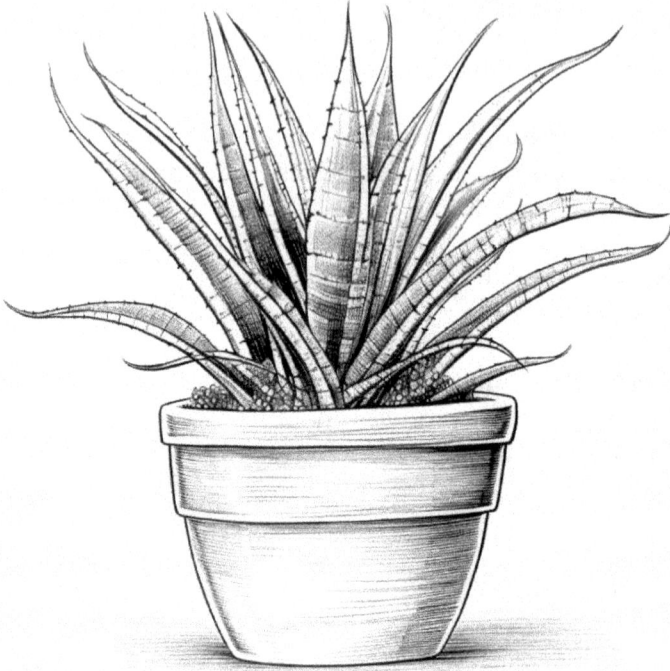

Aloe Vera

- **Healing applications**: sunburn, skin, oral, digestive, and dental health, blood sugar, wound, atopic dermatitis, heartburn, and constipation.

- **Side effects**: Do not take it if you have Crohn's disease, colitis, constipation, or hemorrhoids.

- **Native habitat**: It originated in North Africa but grows well in many U.S. states, including California, Texas, Florida, Arizona, New Mexico, Nevada, Georgia, Louisiana, Alabama, Hawaii, South Carolina, Mississippi, and more.

- **Part(s) used**: fresh leaves

- **Preparation:** Make a tincture, juice, or gel from the fresh leaves.

- **Recommended dosage**: 50 mg daily

- **Application methods**: Add the tincture, juice, or gel to your food, recipes, or drink—or consume them directly.

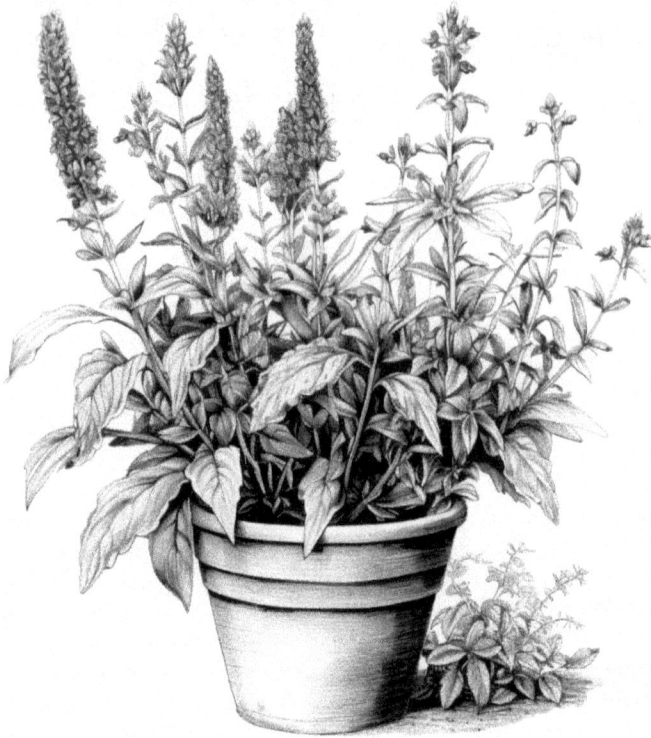

American Skullcap

- **Healing applications**: It is used as a relaxant for anxiety and nervous tension. It improves your mood, reduces inflammation, and is effective against cancer, diarrhea, chronic pain, insomnia, neurodegenerative disease, Alzheimer's, Parkinson's, heart problems, and convulsions.

- **Side effects**: High doses may cause dizziness, liver problems, stupor, twitching, an irregular heartbeat, mental confusion, and seizures. Don't use it if you are pregnant, nursing a baby, or have liver problems. Not safe for children.

- **Native habitat**: You can find this plant in states like Virginia, North Carolina, Maryland, West Virginia, Ohio, Kentucky, Tennessee, Indiana, Illinois, Missouri, Arkansas, and New York.

- **Part(s) used**: 3–4 year plant leaves harvested in June and the plant's roots

- **Preparation**: Grind dried leaves into powder or make tinctures and other liquid forms.

- **Recommended dosage**: 1–2 grams 3 times daily or 240 mL of tea 3 times a day

- **Application methods**: Use it in your recipes, beverages, and for brewing tea.

(*Skullcap Information*, n.d.; Kubala, 2019)

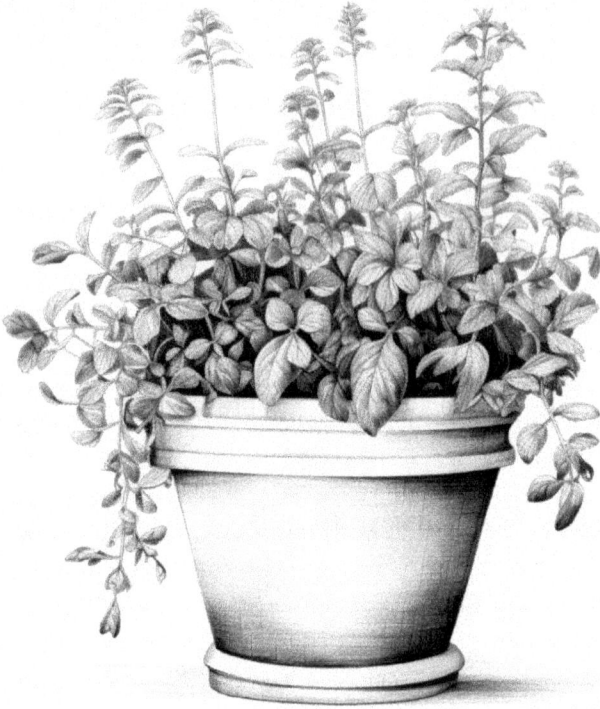

Amla

- **Healing applications**: It is used for reducing anxiety and burning sensations. It is effective for anemic conditions, male infertility, digestive issues, and liver and cardiovascular diseases. Amla is anti-hyperlipidemic, antidiabetic, hypoglycemic, anti-inflammatory, anti-hyperlipidemic, and an antioxidant. This herb is good for mental health, hair growth, eye health, and weight loss.

- **Side effects**: risk of bleeding, reduced sugar levels, dry skin, and aggravated coughing

- **Native habitat**: native to India, Canada, and Southeast Asia.

- **Part(s) used**: Amla is used as a fruit.

- **Preparation**: You can make juice out of amla or eat the fruit directly.

- **Recommended dosage**: This is a fruit you can eat as much as you want.

- **Application methods**: You can consume amla berries fresh or in the form of juices.

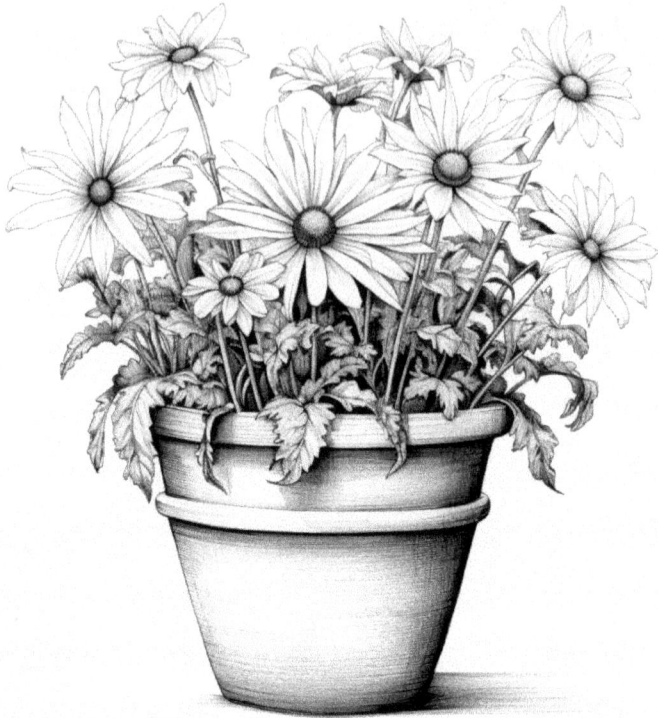

Arnica

- **Healing applications**: It is used to soothe aches, heal wounds, treat superficial phlebitis, and reduce inflammation. You can also use arnica to reduce swelling and treat insect bites, osteoarthritis, and all kinds of external injuries. It shouldn't be taken by mouth except in highly diluted forms.

- **Side effects**: Skin irritation, bleeding, and headaches are some potential side effects.

- **Native habitat**: In America, this herb can be found in states like Montana, Wyoming, Colorado, New Mexico, Arizona, Idaho, Washington, Oregon, California, Nevada, Utah, and North Dakota.

- **Part(s) used**: flowers

- **Preparation**: You should transform it into a cream, tincture, ointment, salve, or lotion.

- **Recommended dosage:** Since it is tagged unsafe by the U.S. Food and Drug Administration, only small amounts are consumed by people or used in pharmaceutical drugs.

- **Application methods**: Use it to brew tea, make tinctures, take in beverages, and apply the oil topically.

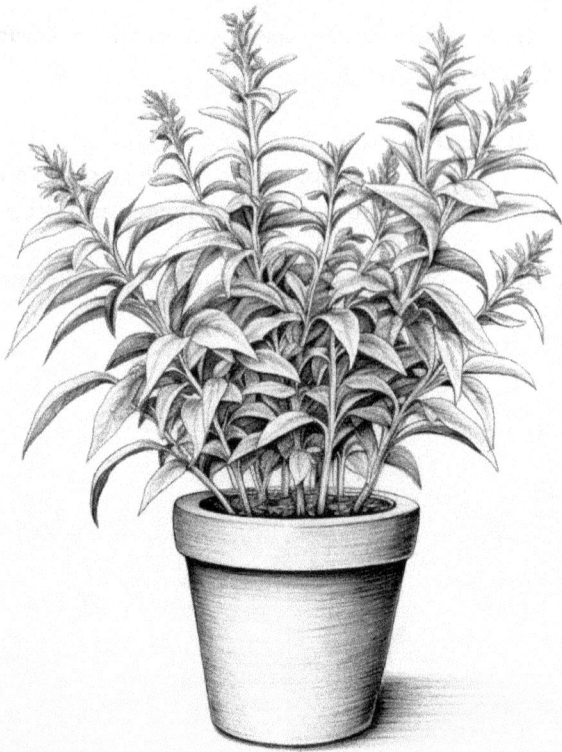

Ashwagandha

- **Healing applications**: It reduces anxiety, supports immunity, decreases cortisol levels, boosts cognitive abilities, improves muscle strength, fights muscle fatigue, alleviates soreness, and improves reproductive health, sleep quality, arthritis symptoms, and blood sugar levels. It is also used for cancer, Alzheimer's, and Parkinson's disease.

- **Side effects**: Ashwagandha can cause miscarriage, sleepiness, slow breathing, increased thyroid levels, and slow the nervous system.

- **Native habitat**: Ashwagandha isn't a domestic plant in the U.S., but it can be cultivated in several states, including California,

Texas, Florida, Arizona, North Carolina, Georgia, New Mexico, Hawaii, Louisiana, Alabama, Mississippi, and others.

- **Part(s) used**: All parts of the plant are used for medicines.

- **Preparation**: You can make it into tinctures, teas, powder, and even creams for topical use.

- **Recommended dosage**: 300 mg to 1000 mg a day is safe for up to 6 months

- **Application methods**: You can consume it alone (it's bitter) or use it for cooking and in your beverages.

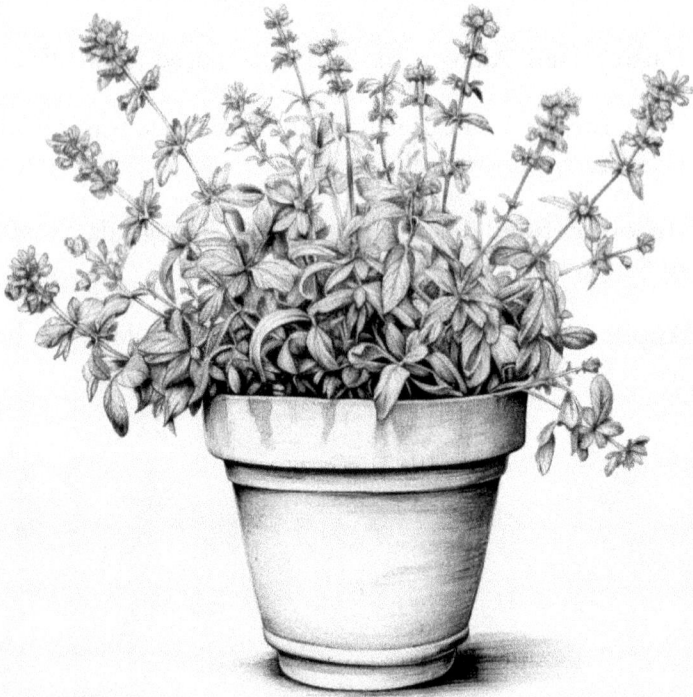

Astragalus

- **Healing applications**: It is effective against cancer and diabetes, supports the immune system to prevent cell damage, and treats colds, upper respiratory infections, and high blood pressure (high BP). It supports the liver, is antibacterial, anti-inflammatory, and a diuretic; is good for skin care and heart disease; lowers cholesterol; alleviates stress, anemia, influenza, fatigue, and lack of appetite. It increases the blood count and treats hepatitis, kidney disease, hay fever, leukemia, and melanoma.

- **Side effects**: It may worsen the cold, cause gastrointestinal discomfort, affect blood pressure levels, cause excessive immune stimulation, stimulate autoimmune responses, affect blood clotting, or cause hormonal interactions.

- **Native habitat**: It is native to Mongolia, China, and Korea. It can be found in several U.S. states, such as Colorado, Arizona, California, Idaho, Montana, Nevada, New Mexico, Oregon, Utah, and others.

- **Part(s) used**: Harvest the roots of 4-year-old plants or older.

- **Preparation:** capsules, powders, tinctures, and teas

- **Recommended dosage**: 500–1,500 mg of the powder daily

- **Application methods**: **and** You can brew tea, make capsules from the powder, or add it to your food and beverages.

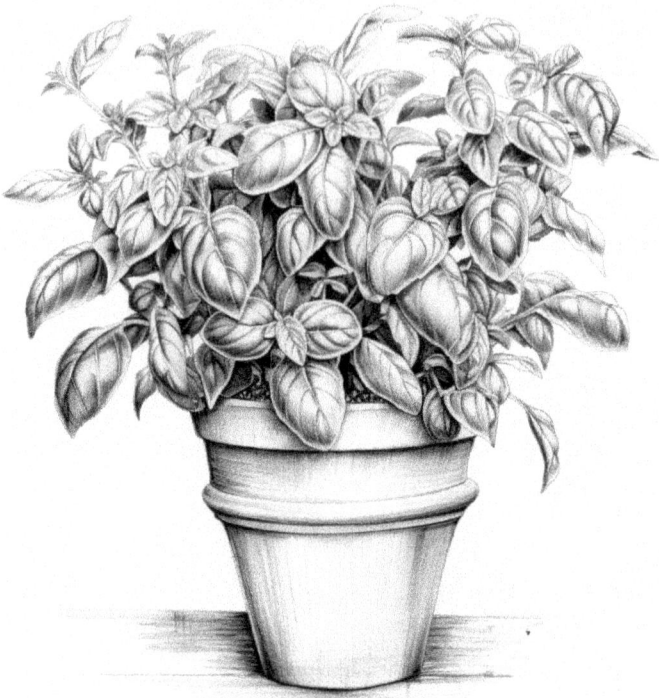

Basil

- **Healing applications**: It is used to reduce oxidative stress and treat cancer, heart disease, diabetes, and arthritis. It can also improve blood flow and reduce cholesterol and inflammation. You can use Holy Basil for skin, urinary, abdominal, and respiratory infections. Holy basil is an antibacterial agent that increases T-cells for better immunity. People also use it to treat asthma, depression, mental health, and memory loss.

- **Side effects**: It may lower blood sugar, impact reproductive hormones, cause digestive issues, undermine blood clotting, impact liver function, and interfere with some medications.

- **Native habitat**: Native to India, Asia, and Africa. It is available in several states, such as California, Texas, Florida, New York, Georgia, and Arizona.

- **Part(s) used**: leaves, stems, and seeds, with fresh leaves for best results.

- **Preparation**: Basil is typically used fresh or processed into essential oil. You can make teas, tinctures, powders, and essential oil from Holy Basil.

- **Recommended dosage**: 300 to 600 mg powder extract or 2–3 cups of tea daily

- **Application methods**: You may also dry and grind it. You can use the plant in cooking or add it to your drinks and snacks.

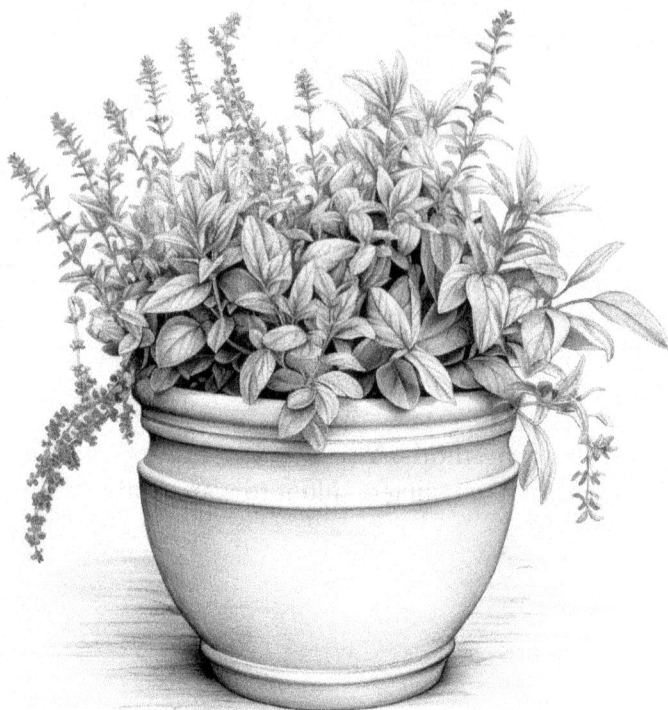

Berberine

- **Healing applications**: This plant is used to treat diabetes, high blood pressure, obesity, heart conditions, gut issues, pneumonia, meningitis, prostate cancer, lung cancer, ovarian cancer, cervical cancer, and liver cancer. It is antimicrobial, antibacterial, and anti-inflammatory, which helps with weight loss, cholesterol, and fertility. This herb contains some of the best cancer-fighting agents, with researchers saying it is highly effective against various cancers.

- **Side effects**: It may cause an upset stomach, constipation, nausea, headache, muscle tremor, gastric ulcers, liver and kidney enlargement, and reduction in white blood cells.

- **Native habitat**: This plant is native to North America and other countries. You can source it from many states, like Oregon, Washington, California, Idaho, Montana, Utah, and Colorado.

- **Part(s) used**: roots, rhizomes, and bark

- **Preparation**: capsules, tablets, tinctures, and creams

- **Recommended dosage**: 900 to 1500 mg per day

- **Application methods**: It is typically used as a cream or orally ingested with food to enhance absorption.

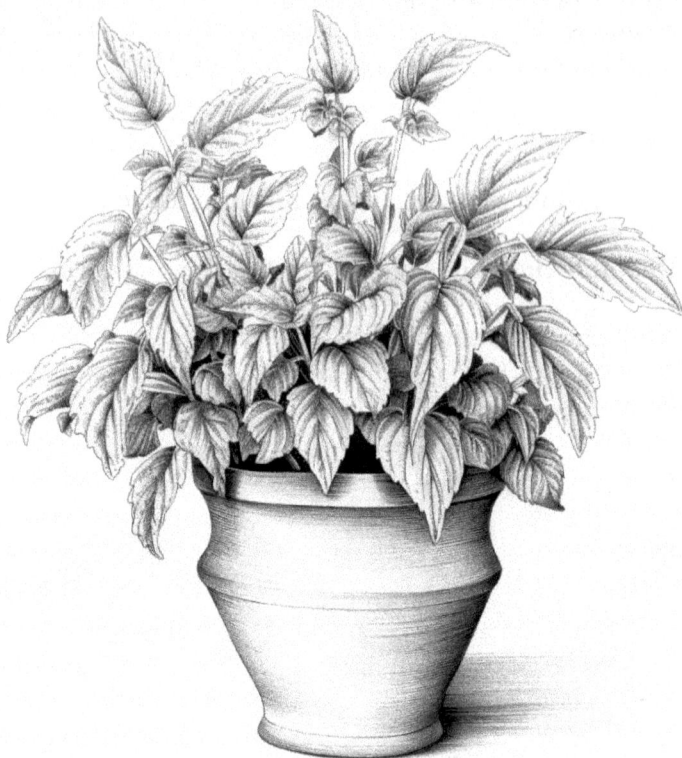

Black Cohosh

- **Healing applications**: It has been used for centuries to treat menstrual issues, fever, musculoskeletal pain, pneumonia, cough, sluggish labor, reproductive problems, vaginal dryness, sleep apnea, vertigo, heart palpitations, tinnitus, and irritability. It increases female fertility, shrinks fibroids, and improves mental health.

- **Side effects**: Do not take Black Cohosh if you have liver disease, as it may cause liver damage or anemia.

- **Native habitat**: This plant is native to North America and grows in West Virginia, Ohio, Kentucky, Tennessee, Georgia, North Carolina, Maryland, Pennsylvania, and other states.

- **Part(s) used**: rhizome and roots

- **Preparation**: capsules, tablets, tinctures, and teas

- **Recommended dosage**: Anything from 20–120 mg of powder is safe.

- **Application methods**: It is taken in hot water, tea, and other beverages.

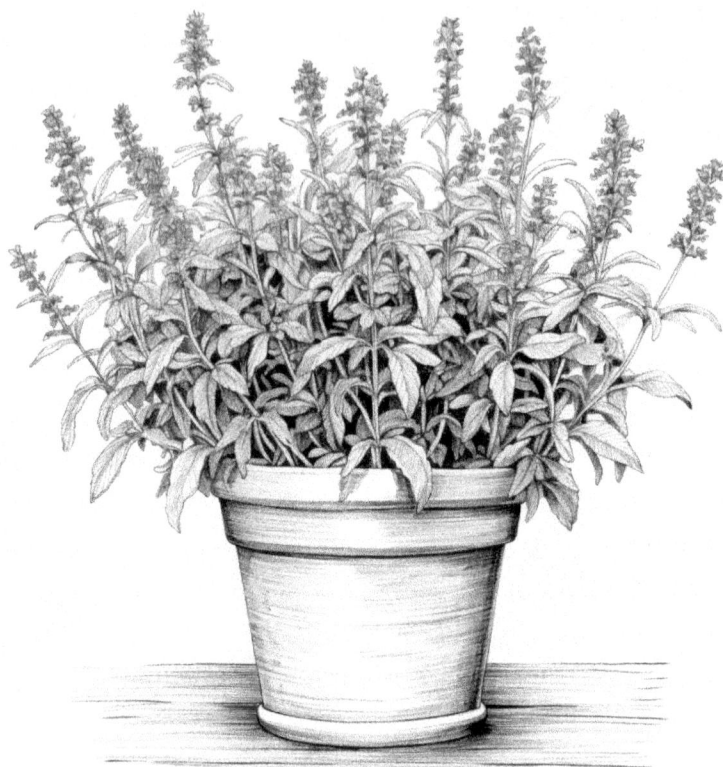

Black Cumin

- **Healing applications**: People use the seed to treat airway disorders, chronic headaches, back pain, diabetes, paralysis, inflammation, bacterial infection, hypertension, digestive issues, neurological or mental illnesses, cancer, infertility, cardiovascular conditions, viral and fungal infections, ulcers, arthritis, coughing, high blood pressure, hypertension, kidney stones, allergies, and rhinitis. It is also used topically for eczema, blisters, swollen joints, orchitis, and nasal abscesses. This herb is good for pregnant, breastfeeding, and menstruating women. It alleviates breast pain, increases breast milk, sperm count, and motility, causes seizures, causes hepatitis, and can cause weight loss.

- **Side effects**: It may increase the risk of breast cancer, digestive upset, nausea, skin rashes, infection, muscle pain, and breast enlargement.

- **Native habitat**: It is available in many U.S. states, such as California, Texas, Florida, New York, Arizona, Illinois, Ohio, North Carolina, and Pennsylvania.

- **Part(s) used**: roots and rhizomes

- **Preparation**: Dig up the roots and rhizomes and make them into powders, infusions, and tinctures.

- **Recommended dosage**: 500 mg to 2,000 mg of oil or powder daily

- **Application methods**: Use the powder and oil in your food and beverages.

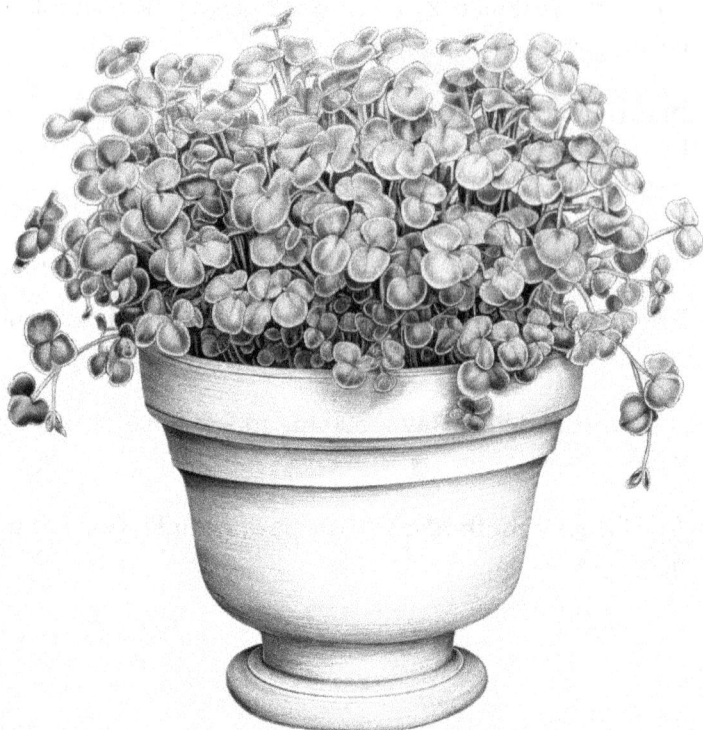

Brahmi

- **Healing applications**: It is an anxiolytic used to treat insomnia, memory improvement, anxiety, cognitive enhancement, attention deficit hyperactivity disorder (ADHD) symptoms, inflammation, stress, anxiety, cancer, heart disease, diabetes, kidney disease, brain function, impulsivity, inattentiveness, moodiness, high BP, breast, pain relief, and colon cancer.

- **Side effects**: intestinal cramps, increased stool frequency, diarrhea, and nausea. It's not recommended for pregnant or lactating women.

- **Native habitat**: It can be found in Florida, Texas, California, Arizona, Georgia, North Carolina, Louisiana, and Hawaii.

- **Part(s) used**: leaves, stems, and roots.

- **Preparation**: Dry and grind these parts into powder or make a tincture, oil, tea, or infusions from them.

- **Recommended dosage**: 300 to 600 mg daily

- **Application methods**: You can take the herbal preparations in water, food, or beverages.

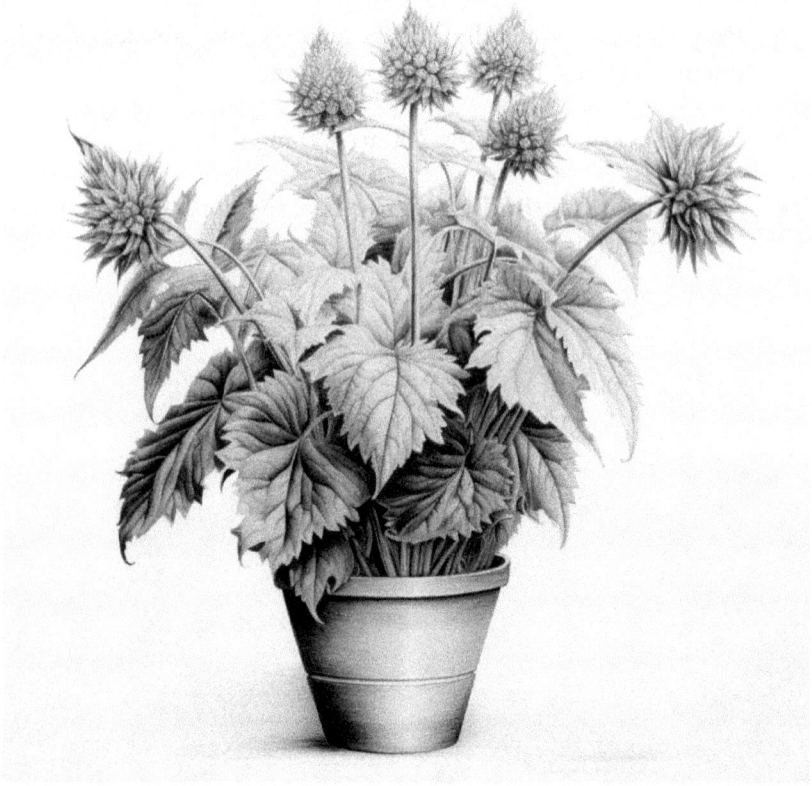

Burdock

- **Healing applications**: Packed with powerful antioxidants, it is used to treat inflammation, purify the blood, increase sexual function, ease acne and eczema, and treat burns.

- **Side effects**: Adverse reactions include skin irritation, anaphylaxis, shortness of breath, swelling, constipation, diarrhea, stomach upset, bloating, and low blood sugar. Be careful when harvesting or buying burdock because you can easily mix or confuse it with belladonna nightshade, a close look-alike that is highly toxic and usually grows together. The plant's roots are used as a diuretic and can cause dehydration. Not recommended for pregnant women or those who want to conceive a baby.

- **Native habitat**: This plant is native to Europe and North Asia but is now grown in U.S. states like New York, Pennsylvania, California, Michigan, Illinois, Ohio, Texas, Wisconsin, and Massachusetts.

- **Part(s) used**: fresh or dried roots and seeds

- **Preparation**: capsules, tinctures, teas, and poultices

- **Recommended dosage**: 2–6 grams powder or 1–2 mL of tincture daily

- **Application methods**: You can use the fresh roots for tea or dry and grind it into powder for use in cooking.

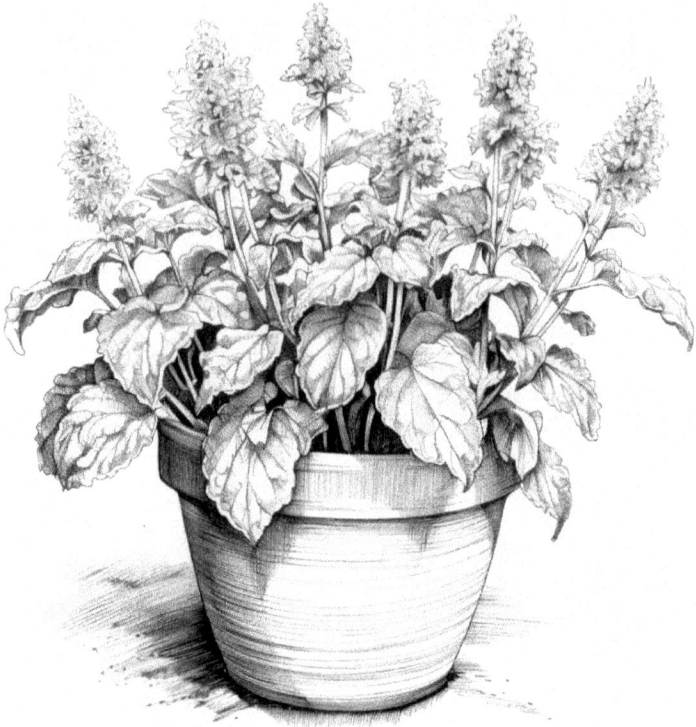

Butterbur

- **Healing applications**: It is used for spasms, swelling, asthma, migraine, hay fever, upset stomach, allergies, wounds, cough, and urinary tract infections.

- **Side effects**: If excessively used, it may cause liver problems, belching, drowsiness, fatigue, diarrhea, itching eyes, and stomach upset. Some butterbur products are contaminated with pyrrolizidine alkaloids (PAs), which can damage the liver and lungs.

- **Native habitat**: You can find this herb in New York, Pennsylvania, California, Michigan, Illinois, Ohio, Texas, Wisconsin, Massachusetts, and other states.

- **Part(s) used**: roots and seeds

- **Preparation**: You can make tinctures, juices, gels, and powders from this plant.

- **Recommended dosage**: 10–180 mg daily for 16 weeks

- **Application methods**: You can take it orally in water, beverages, or tea.

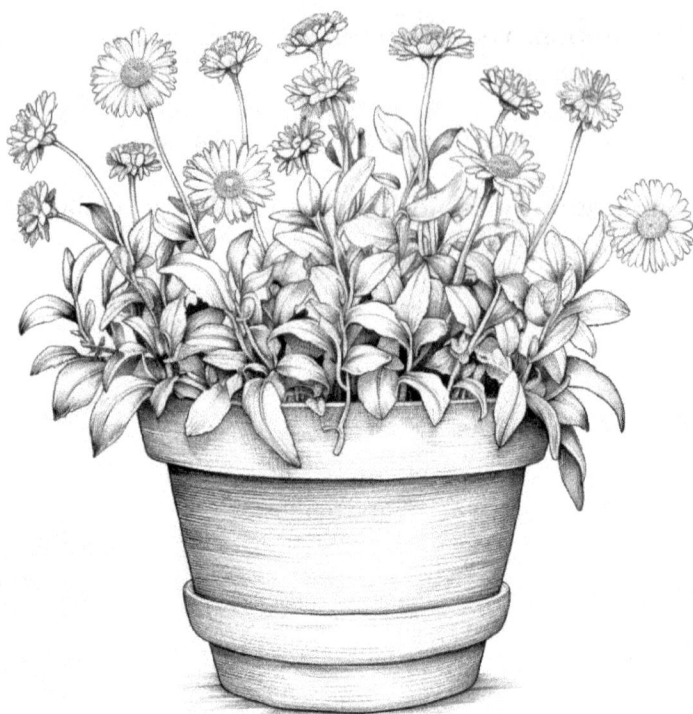

Calendula

- **Healing applications**: It is used for inflammation, bacterial and viral infections, ulcers, insomnia, fever, stress, stomach upset, menstrual cramps, and topically for wounds, hemorrhoids, diaper rash, ear infection, and skin health. Calendula helps prevent dermatitis during cancer treatment by radiation. It is particularly effective in quick healing of wounds.

- **Side effects**: This herb may impact the liver, upset stomach, cause diarrhea, affect blood pressure levels, increase sensitivity to sunlight, cause weight gain, and interact with certain drugs.

- **Native habitat**: It originates from Mediterranean countries but now grows throughout the world. You can also find it in

California, Texas, New York, Pennsylvania, Florida, Ohio, Illinois, Michigan, Massachusetts, and other locations.

- **Part(s) used**: rhizomes and leaves

- **Preparation**: You can make creams, infusions, tinctures, wound washes, ointments, and powders from the dried petals.

- **Recommended dosage**: 50–100 mg daily

- **Application methods**: You can take it orally in beverages or foods. Use it topically as a mouthwash or for sore nipples.

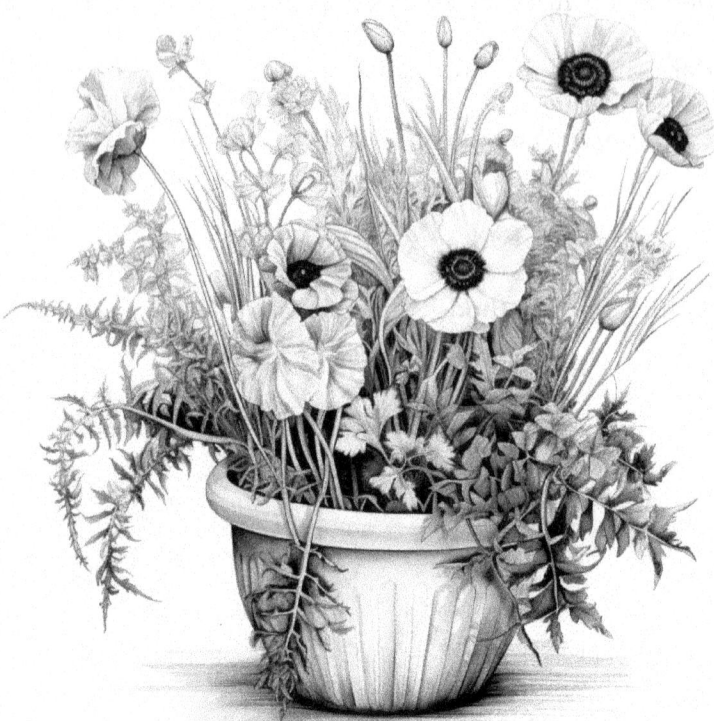

California Poppy

- **Healing applications**: It is used for headaches, muscle pain, anxiety, stress, cough, respiratory illnesses, urinary tract infections, high BP, toothaches, nerve pain, inflammations, mental health, digestive issues, and menstrual cramps.

- **Side effects**: drowsiness, nausea, stomach upset, itching, rash, and swelling.

- **Native habitat**: This plant originated in Mexico and the western United States. It can be found in California, Nevada, Washington, Oregon, and other states.

- **Part(s) used**: Harvest the aerial parts, such as leaves, flowers, and stems, when the plant blooms.

- **Preparation**: You can make a tincture, essential oil, powder, or tea with the leaves, flowers, and stems of this plant.

- **Recommended dosage**: The recommended dosage ranges from 10–20 tincture drops or a cup of California Poppy tea daily.

- **Application methods**: Use it in teas, foods, beverages, and other edibles.

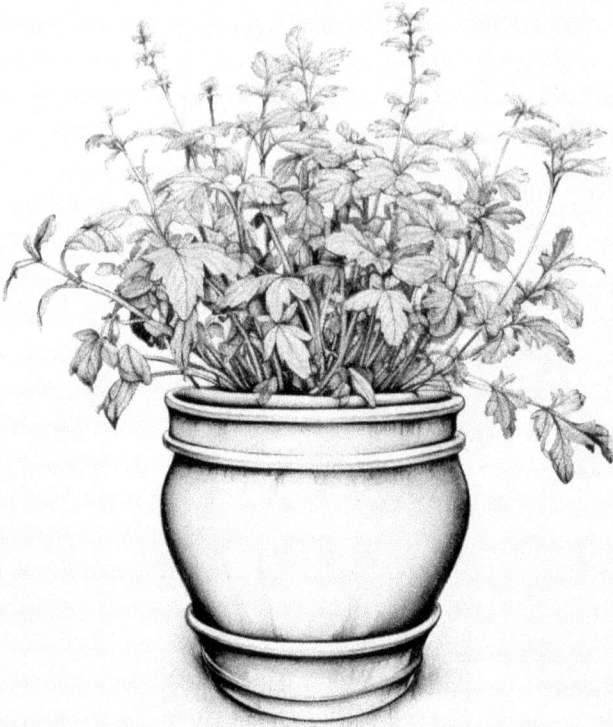

Caraway

- **Healing applications**: It is used for digestive health, bloating and gas, colic in infants, spasms, low appetite, inflammations, respiratory health, menstrual pain, boosting breast milk, coughs, bronchitis, sleep quality, weight loss, and more.

- **Side effects**: itching, rash, swelling, bloating, gas, skin redness, and irritation.

- **Native habitat**: This plant originated in North Africa, Europe, and Western Asia. In America, it grows in North Dakota and Michigan, among others.

- **Part(s) used**: Harvest and dry the umbels, and then use the seeds.

- **Preparation**: Make some tea, infusions, tinctures, powder, or essential oil from the seeds.

- **Recommended dosage**: 1–2 teaspoons of crushed seed in a cup of tea, or 0.1–0.9 grams of Caraway essential oil daily.

- **Application methods**: You can take your preparations in tea, food, beverages, or snacks.

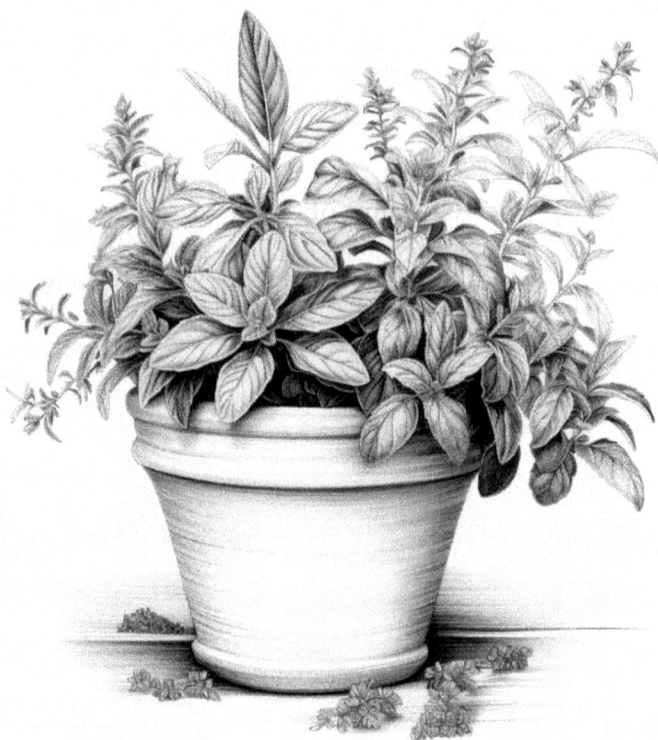

Cardamon

- **Healing applications**: It can be used for indigestion, bad breath, respiratory problems, inflammations, high BP, liver health, moodiness, bacterial infections, muscle pain, oral health, nausea, nasal congestion, arthritis, cardiovascular health, immune health, sexual wellness, and kidney function.

- **Side effects**: skin rash, itching, diarrhea, stomach upset, lower BP, dizziness, lightheadedness, and weakened blood clothing.

- **Native habitat**: It is native to Asian countries like India, Guatemala, and Sri Lanka. It can also be found in Florida, Hawaii, and California.

- **Part(s) used**: seeds

- **Preparation**: You can make tinctures, essential oils, powders, and infusions from the seeds.

- **Recommended dosage**: 1–2 teaspoons of powder or 0.1–0.5 grams of essential oil a day

- **Application methods**: Use it in your beverages or tea.

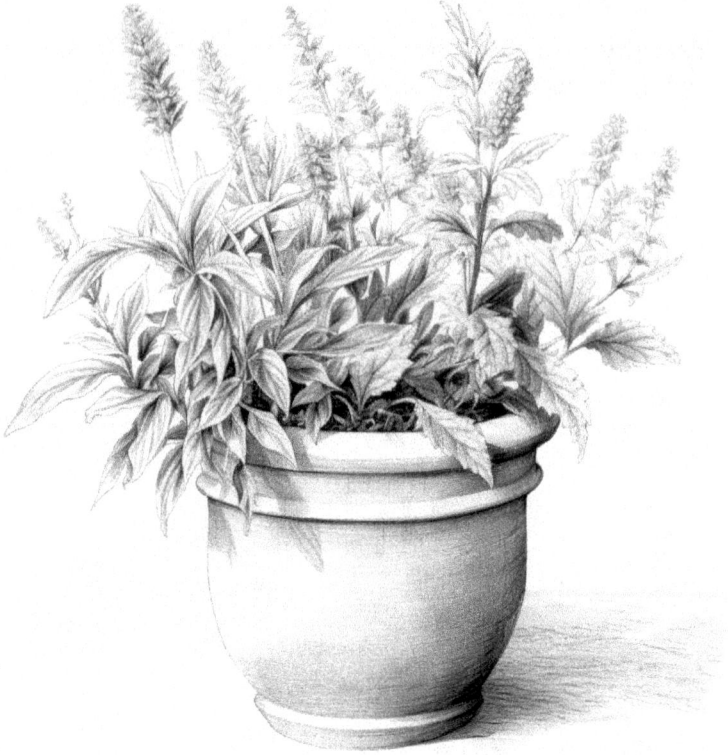

Cat's Claw

- **Healing applications**: Use this plant to boost the immune system, cure arthritis, manage stress, treat gastritis, relieve joint pain, and treat viral infections like herpes. It can also be used for bacterial infections, cancer prevention, cardiovascular health, high blood pressure, cognitive function, anxiety, and Lyme disease.

- **Side effects**: Potential adverse reactions include dizziness, diarrhea, lower blood pressure, skin rash, itching, and autoimmune disorders.

- **Native habitat**: It is native to the Amazon rainforest and grows in states like Hawaii, Texas, Louisiana, New York, and others.

- **Part(s) used**: inner bark and root

- **Preparation**: powder, tinctures, teas, and infusions.

- **Recommended dosage**: 1–2 mg daily

- **Application methods**: brewed as tea or taken as capsules

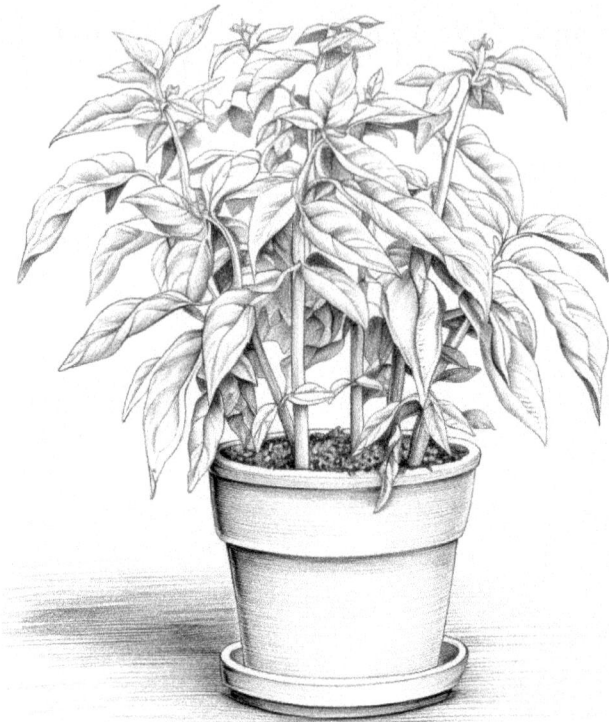

Cayenne

- **Healing applications**: It is used for migraines, joint pain, bloating and gas, cardiovascular health, heart health, arthritis, weight loss, muscle and nerve pain, high blood pressure, cold and flu, cancer, fast wound healing, bleeding, ulcers, bacterial infections, and nerve health.

- **Side effects**: Potential adverse reactions include stomach irritation, diarrhea, capsaicin sensitivity, and liver and kidney damage.

- **Native habitat**: It originates from Central and South America and is available in North Carolina, New Mexico, Arizona, Texas, Louisiana, and other states.

- **Part(s) used**: fruits and seeds

- **Preparation**: tinctures, powders, creams, and capsules

- **Recommended dosage**: 30–120 mg of powder daily or 0.3–1.5 ml for tinctures

- **Application methods**: It is used orally for internal problems or topically for pain relief.

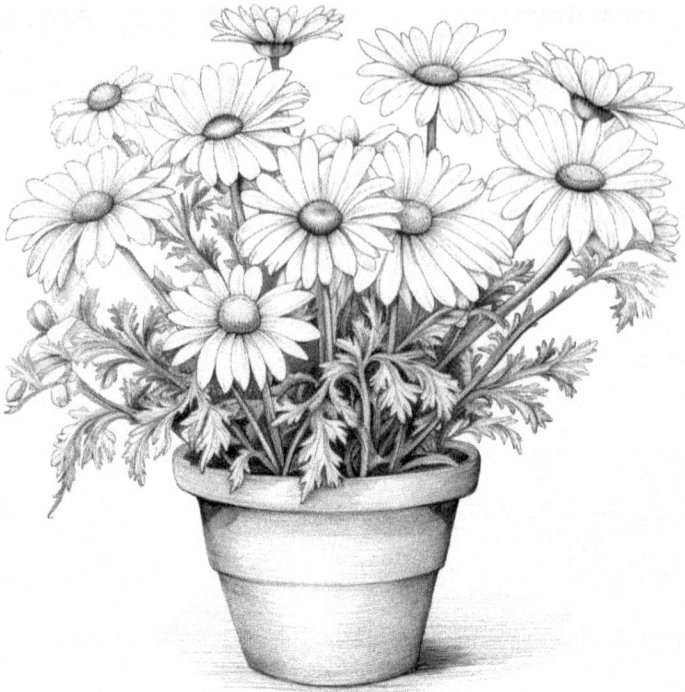

Chamomile

- **Healing applications**: It is used to ease indigestion, bloating, insomnia, stress, anxiety, skin inflammation, eczema, menstrual cramps, congestion, sore throats, and bacterial infections. It can also boost the immune system, calm nerves, alleviate IBS, manage diabetes, prevent cancer, improve scalp health, and kill dandruff.

- **Side effects**: As a result of using this herb, you may experience rash or itching, uterine stimulation, cross-reactivity, undermining of blood-thinning medications, eye irritation, nausea, vomiting, and eczema aggravation in some people.

- **Native habitat**: It originated in Europe and Western Asia but also grows in Oregon, Michigan, Ohio, Texas, Pennsylvania, and other states.

- **Part(s) used**: flowers

- **Preparation**: tea, capsules, powder, essential oil, tincture, and infusions.

- **Recommended dosage**: 1–2 teaspoons of dried flower powder in tea or 1–4 grams of dried flower daily.

- **Application methods**: You should take it as tea or apply it topically for skin health.

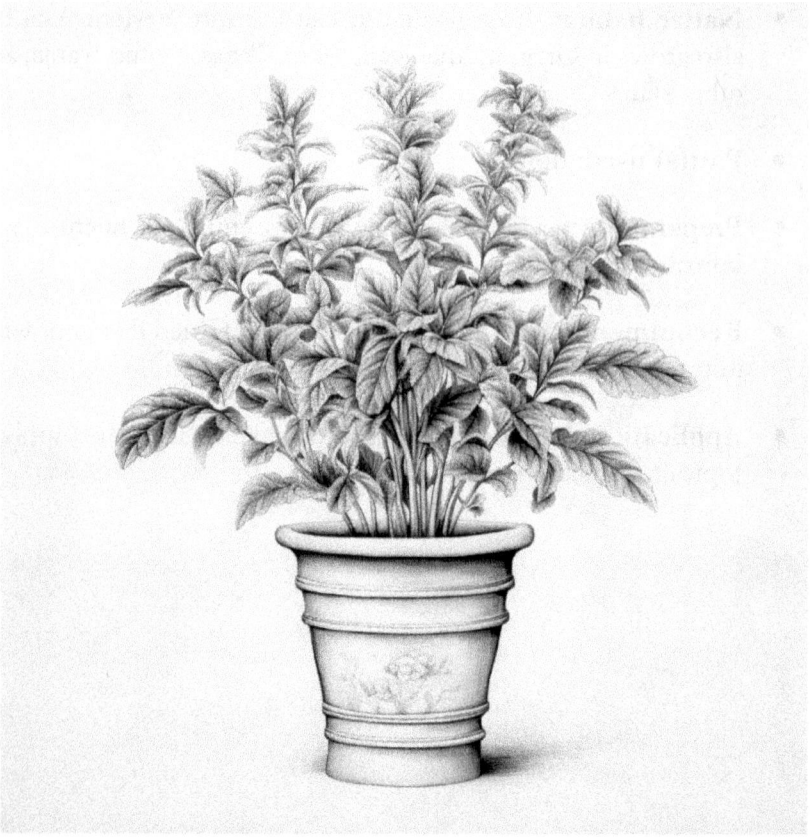

Chaste Tree

- **Healing applications**: It eases PMS and endometriosis symptoms, alleviates hot flashes, regulates menstrual cycles, prevents mood swings, enhances fertility, reduces hormonal acne in women, and eases mastalgia. It can also help with uterine fibroids, low sex drive, anxiety, indigestion, migraine, arthritis, weight loss, insomnia, and Polycystic Ovary Syndrome (PCO) support.

- **Side effects**: digestive discomfort, headaches, skin rash, itching, hormonal imbalance, dizziness, weight changes, and strong sex drive.

- **Native habitat**: It originated in the Mediterranean region and is now cultivated in Virginia, Georgia, California, Texas, New York, Ohio, Pennsylvania, and Florida.

- **Part(s) used**: fruit

- **Preparation**: dried fruit extracts, tinctures, and capsules

- **Recommended dosage**: 40 drops of tincture or 20–40 mg of dried fruit extract daily.

- **Application methods**: taken orally as tinctures or capsules, or consumed as fruits

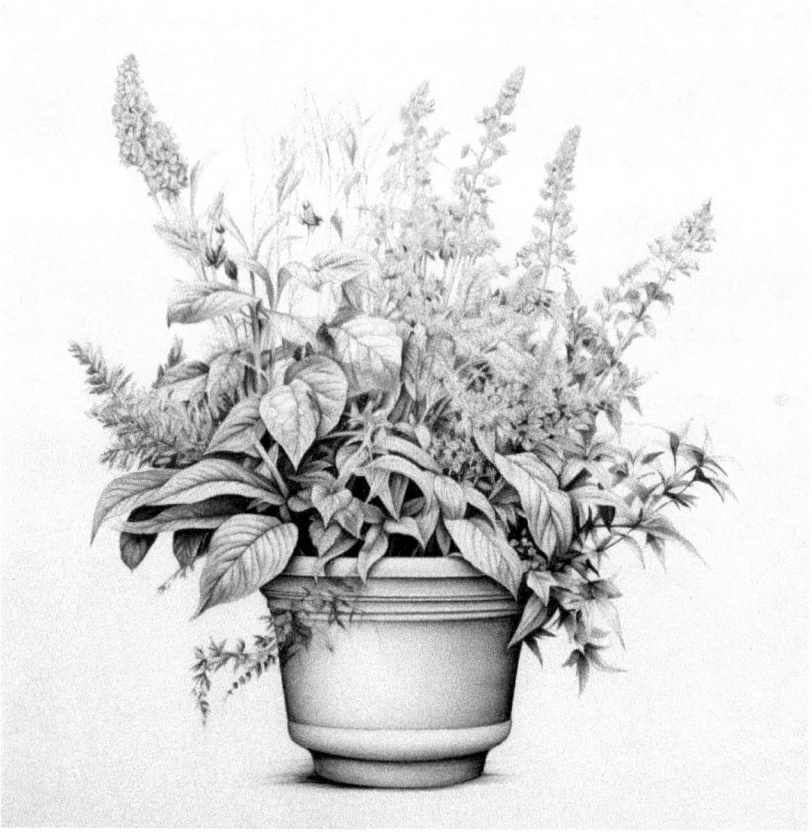

Chinese Skullcap

- **Healing applications**: Chinese skullcap has anti-cancer properties and can treat conditions like liver disease, diarrhea, gastrointestinal issues, insomnia, fevers, dysentery, inflammation, high BP, respiratory infections, hepatitis, and hemorrhaging.

- **Side effects**: It may lower blood sugar levels. Avoid it if you have spleen or stomach problems.

- **Native habitat**: It is native to China, Russia, and other Asian countries but also grows in states like California, Oregon, Washington, Nevada, Arizona, New Mexico, Texas, Florida, Georgia, North Carolina, and more.

- **Part(s) used**: collect the leaves and roots of the plant.

- **Preparation:** Make a tincture or juice from the fresh leaves and roots, or make powders from the dried form.

- **Recommended dosage**: 1–2 grams 3 times daily or 240 mL of tea 3 times a day

- **Application methods**: Use this herb to brew tea and make tinctures, infusions, juices, or other beverages.

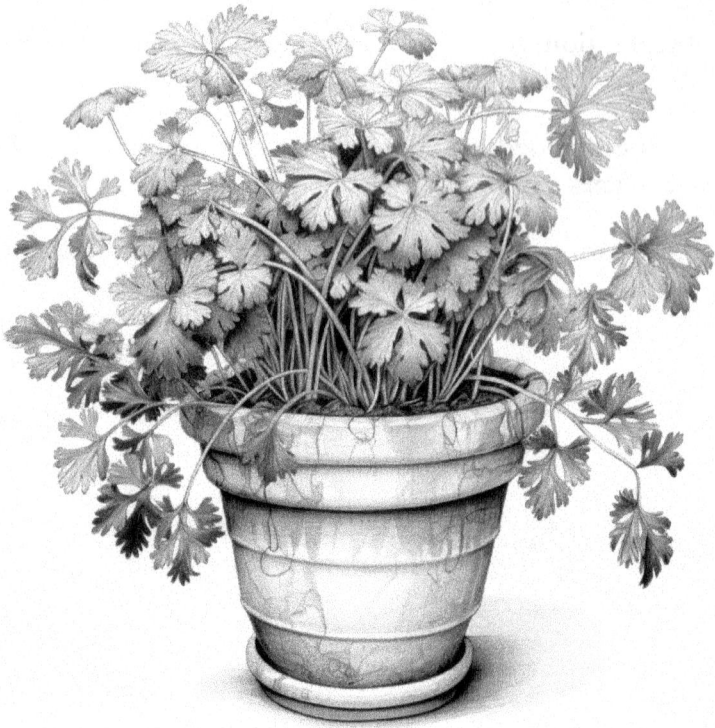

Cilantro

- **Healing applications**: Use this plant to detoxify the body, ease digestion, treat arthritis and bloating, alleviate stress, lower cholesterol, and regulate blood sugar levels. It can also support the immune system, kill bacteria, reduce bad breath, treat oral infections, and manage anxiety. It is great for bone health, stress, cancer prevention, and eye and bone health.

- **Side effects**: skin irritation, excesses may cause digestive issues, lower blood pressure, impact hormonal levels, and sensitivity to light

- **Native habitat**: Its origin traces back to the Mediterranean region but is currently obtainable in Colorado, California, New Mexico, Illinois, Texas, Arizona, Georgia, and Florida.

- **Part(s) used**: leaves and seeds

- **Preparation:** You can make tinctures, capsules, essential oils, and powder from the fresh or dried leaves of cilantro.

- **Recommended dosage**: 1–3 grams of dried leaves or seeds daily

- **Application methods**: Use it in your tea, beverages, culinary dishes, and other edibles.

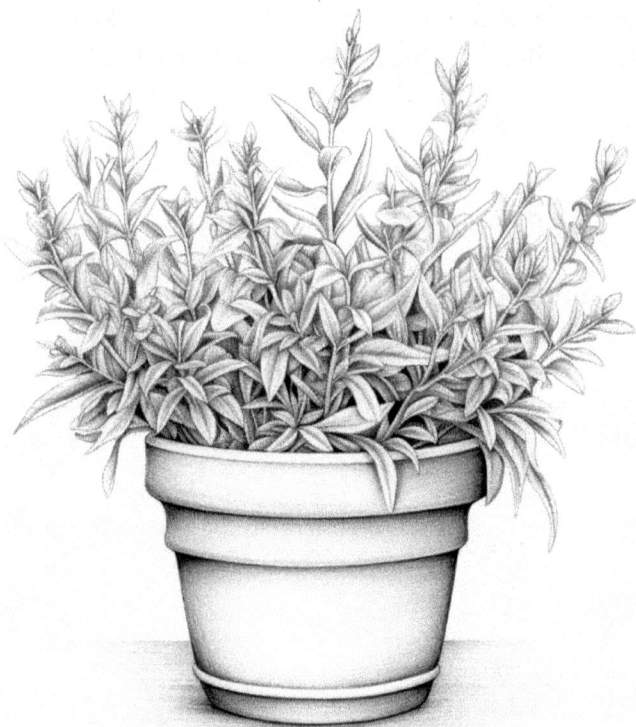

Cinnamon

- **Healing applications**: It is used to regulate blood sugar, reduce inflammation, manage stress, and support heart health. You can also use this herb to lower cholesterol levels, ease digestion and bloating, treat bacterial infections, lose weight, relieve arthritis, enhance cognitive abilities, prevent cancer, and provide menstrual pain relief. Other uses include improving respiratory health and preventing moodiness.

- **Side effects**: Excessive consumption may cause liver damage, interfere with diabetic and high-BP medications, cause digestive issues, and pose a risk to pregnant women.

- **Native habitat**: It is available in several U.S. states, including Mississippi, Louisiana, California, Hawaii, Texas, South and North Carolina, and Georgia.

- **Part(s) used**: bark

- **Preparation**: dried and ground, essential oil, powder, capsule, and tea.

- **Recommended dosage**: 0.05–0.2 ml of its oil, or 1–6 grams of cinnamon powder.

- **Application methods**: Take cinnamon orally in tea, beverages, or foods.

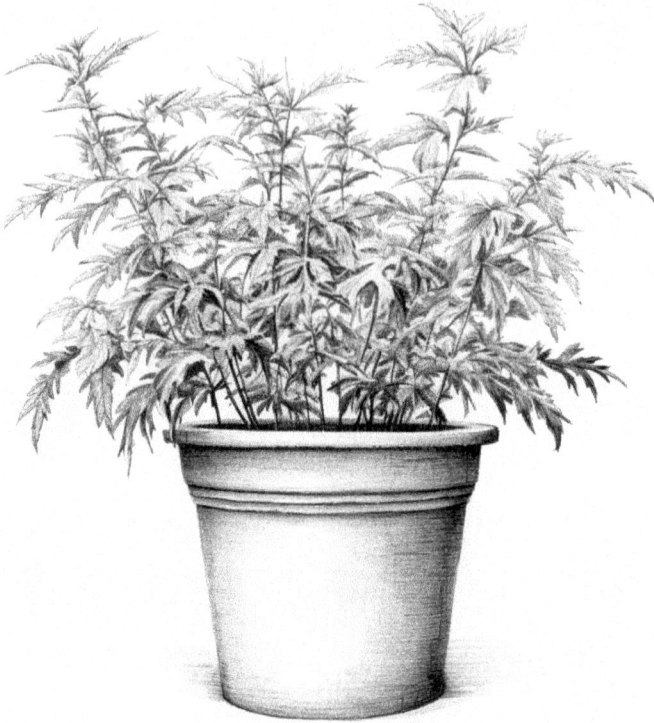

Cleavers

- **Healing applications**: This plant is known to treat lymphatic congestion, enhance urine flow and detoxification, treat eczema and psoriasis, joint inflammation, urinary tract infections, heal wounds, purify the blood, and prevent cancer. You can also use it against bloating and gas, fever, respiratory illnesses, and arthritis. It supports the liver and balances hormones.

- **Side effects**: skin rash and itching, digestive issues, sensitivity to light, interference with BP medications, stomach irritation, and may impact kidney function.

- **Native habitat**: It is native to North America, Europe, and Asia, and can be found in several U.S. states, such as Michigan,

Oregon, California, Pennsylvania, Illinois, New York, Texas, Florida, and Washington.

- **Part(s) used**: leaves, stems, and flowers

- **Preparation**: teas, capsules, powder, tinctures, essential oils, and infusions

- **Recommended dosage**: 20–40 drops of tincture or 2–4 grams of powder.

- **Application methods**: You can take it in food, beverages, tea, or topically apply it on the skin.

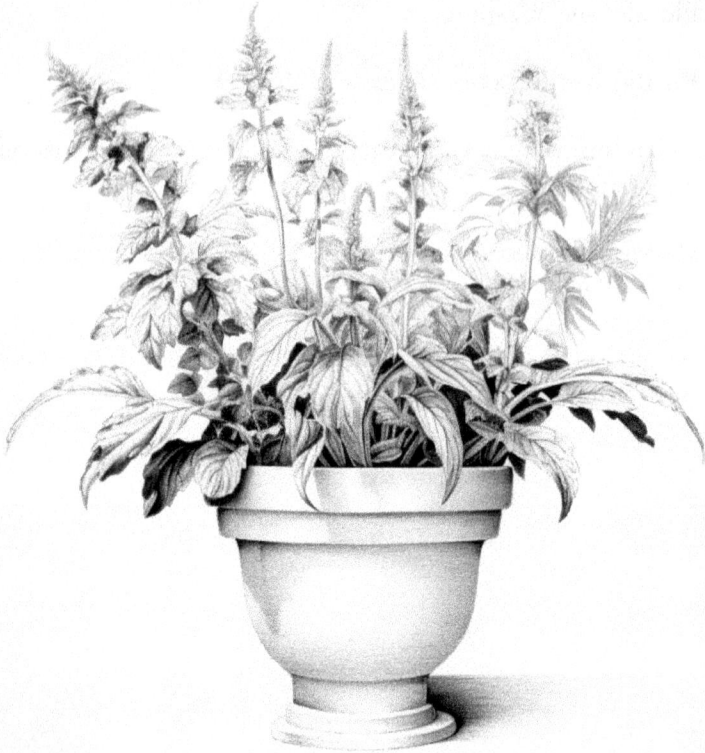

Codonopsis

- **Healing applications**: helps the body adapt to stress, enhances immune function, combats physical and mental fatigue, alleviates respiratory issues, aids in managing blood sugar levels, eases digestive discomfort, reduces inflammation, improves blood circulation, addresses anemia-related symptoms, fights oxidative stress, shows potential in cancer prevention, supports heart health, calms the nervous system, supports fertility and reproductive organs, and exhibits antimicrobial properties

- **Side effects**: stomach upset

- **Native habitat**: It is native to East Asian countries and can be found in several U.S. states, including California, Oregon,

Washington, Idaho, Montana, Wyoming, Colorado, Utah, Nevada, Arizona, New Mexico, and Texas.

- **Part(s) used**: roots

- **Preparation**: decoctions, tinctures, powders, and capsules

- **Recommended dosage**: 3–9 grams of dried root daily

- **Application methods**: You can brew this into tea or use it as an ingredient in your recipes.

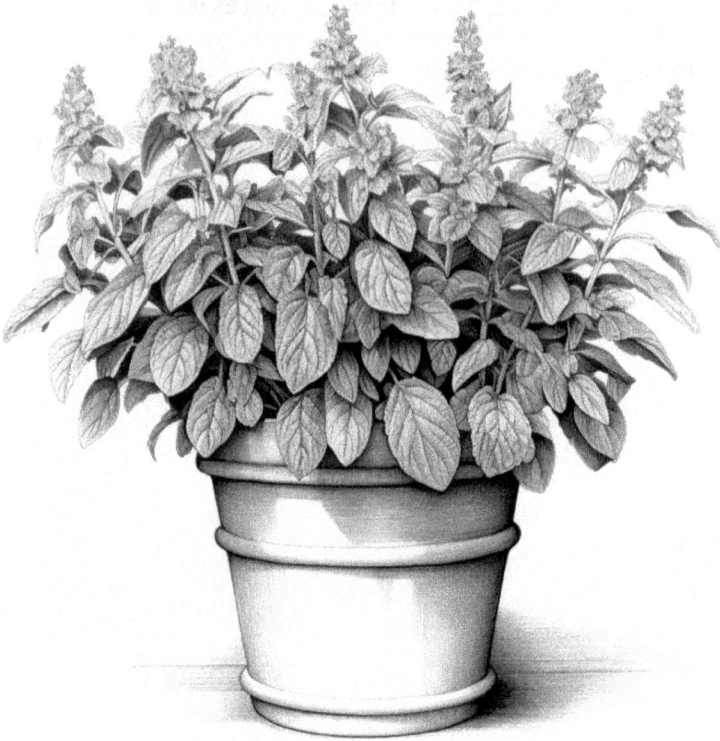

Comfrey

- **Healing applications**: It accelerates healing of cuts and bruises, eases joint pain and inflammation, supports bone healing and density, treats dermatitis, eczema, and psoriasis, alleviates coughs and respiratory issues, relieves symptoms of arthritis, aids in soothing stomach ulcers, used topically for burn recovery, reduces discoloration and pain, eases muscle and joint injuries, treats rough, chapped skin from gardening, assists in soothing gastritis symptoms, eases pain from sprains and strains, reduces discomfort associated with varicose veins, and promotes cell growth for tissue repair.

- **Side effects**: excessive use can cause liver problems

- **Native habitat**: This herb is native to Europe and Asia but can be found in many U.S. states such as California, Oregon, Washington, Idaho, Montana, Wyoming, Colorado, Utah, Nevada, Arizona, New Mexico, Texas, and others.

- **Part(s) used**: leaves and roots

- **Preparation:** ointments, salves, creams, poultices, teas, and capsules

- **Recommended dosage**: We don't recommend orally taking this herb as it contains a dangerous compound, pyrrolizidine alkaloids, which can cause liver problems.

- **Application methods**: It's typically used topically. But if you want to ingest it, consult your doctor first.

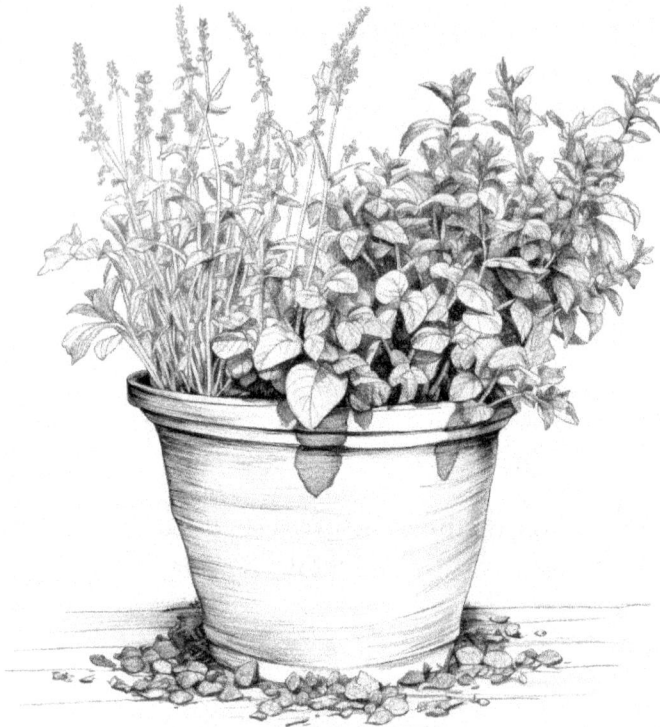

Cramp Bark

- **Healing applications**: It alleviates menstrual cramps and uterine spasms, eases smooth muscle tension during pregnancy, relieves pain associated with menstruation, soothes gastrointestinal spasms, supports bladder function, alleviates arthritic joint pain, assists in bronchial relaxation, aids in reducing blood pressure, calms nervous tension, mitigates tension headaches, acts as a mild sedative, promotes relaxation for better sleep, facilitates uterine recovery after childbirth, relieves symptoms of irritable bowel syndrome, and addresses general muscle cramps and spasms.

- **Side effects**: skin rash or a mild stomach upset

- **Native habitat**: It is native to North America and usually grows in states like New York, Pennsylvania, Ohio, Michigan, and Minnesota.

- **Part(s) used**: bark

- **Preparation**: tinctures, capsules, and teas

- **Recommended dosage**: 1–2 grams of powder or 2–4 mL of tincture thrice a day

- **Application methods**: Brew this herb into tea or take it in hot water after warming it for 10–15 minutes.

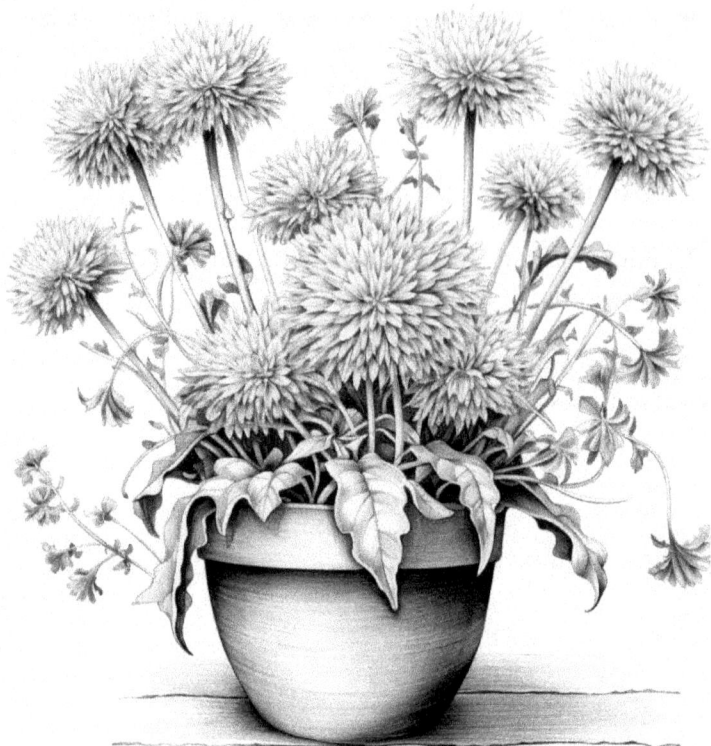

Dandelion

- **Healing applications**: supports liver function and detoxification, eases indigestion and stimulates appetite, promotes kidney health and reduces water retention, aids in managing blood glucose levels, alleviates inflammation in joints, helps maintain healthy cholesterol levels, acts as a natural diuretic for weight management, clears acne and promotes a healthy complexion, enhances immune system function, fights oxidative stress and supports cellular health, assists in maintaining healthy blood pressure, nourishes beneficial gut bacteria, is rich in calcium, supports bone strength, contains compounds with potential anti-cancer properties, and eases respiratory conditions like bronchitis.

- **Side effects**: skin irritation and gastrointestinal upset

- **Native habitat**: You can find this plant in California, Texas, New York, and Illinois.

- **Part(s) used**: leaves, roots, and flowers

- **Preparation**: capsules, tinctures, teas, and powders

- **Recommended dosage**: 500–2000 mg daily

- **Application methods**: Brew a water tea with this herb or steep the leaves and roots in hot water.

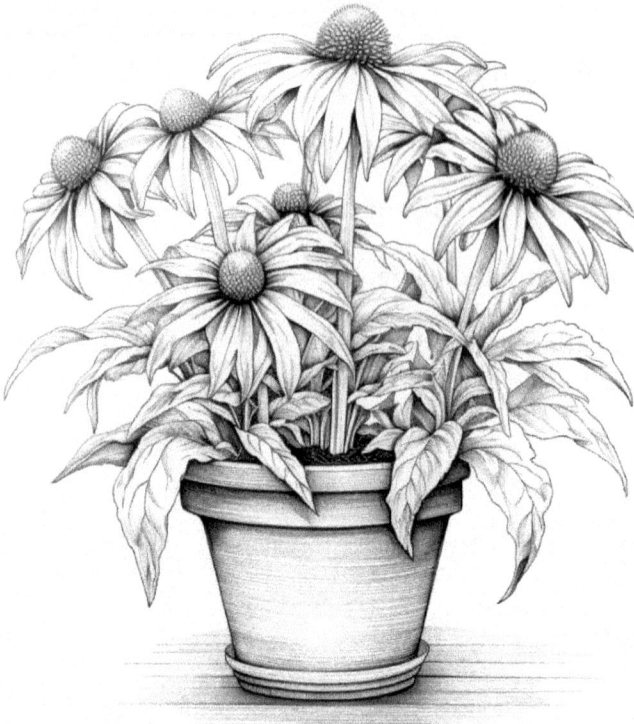

Echinacea

- **Healing applications**: It boosts the immune system to prevent and treat infections, alleviates symptoms of colds, flu, and respiratory infections, reduces inflammation in conditions like arthritis, facilitates the healing of minor wounds and skin conditions, fights viral infections like herpes, combats bacterial infections, mitigates symptoms of hay fever and allergies, supports the treatment of UTIs, eases symptoms of gingivitis and oral infections, exhibits potential anti-cancer properties, acts as a mild pain reliever for conditions like headaches, treats skin conditions such as eczema, may alleviate symptoms of anxiety and depression, improves lymphatic circulation, and aids in promoting a healthy appetite.

- **Side effects**: skin rash, upset stomach, gastrointestinal issues with doses.

- **Native habitat**: This herb is native to North America and can be found in states like Kansas, Oklahoma, Nebraska, and Texas.

- **Part(s) used**: roots, leaves, and flowers

- **Preparation**: powder, capsules, tinctures, teas, and creams

- **Recommended dosage**: 300–500 mg powder or 1–2 grams of dried herb

- **Application methods**: Add the tincture or powder to your beverages and recipes or brew it into tea.

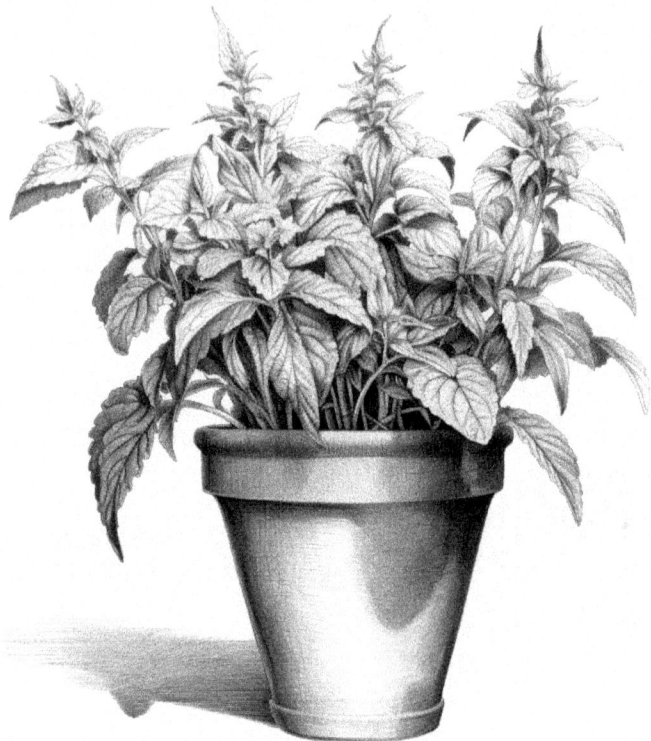

Elder

- **Healing applications**: It enhances the immune system to prevent illness, fights viral infections, including influenza, eases symptoms of colds, flu, and bronchitis, reduces inflammation in arthritis and joint pain, lowers fever associated with infections, promotes kidney health and reduces water retention, alleviates constipation and indigestion, soothes coughs and throat irritation, treats wounds, burns, and eczema, is rich in antioxidants, promotes skin health, mitigates symptoms of allergies, supports heart health, aids in preventing urinary tract infections, relieves occasional constipation, and helps regulate blood sugar levels.

- **Side effects**: nausea, diarrhea, itching, or skin rashes

- **Native habitat**: It is native to North America and grows in several states, including but not limited to California, New York, Texas, and Florida.

- **Part(s) used**: flowers, berries, and bark

- **Preparation**: syrups, powders, teas, capsules, and tinctures

- **Recommended dosage**: 1–2 teaspoons of syrup, 2–3 grams of dried parts, or 300–500 mg of pure extracts

- **Application methods**: You can take the syrup alone or in a beverage. The dried parts can be used to brew tea, or you can take the capsules with water.

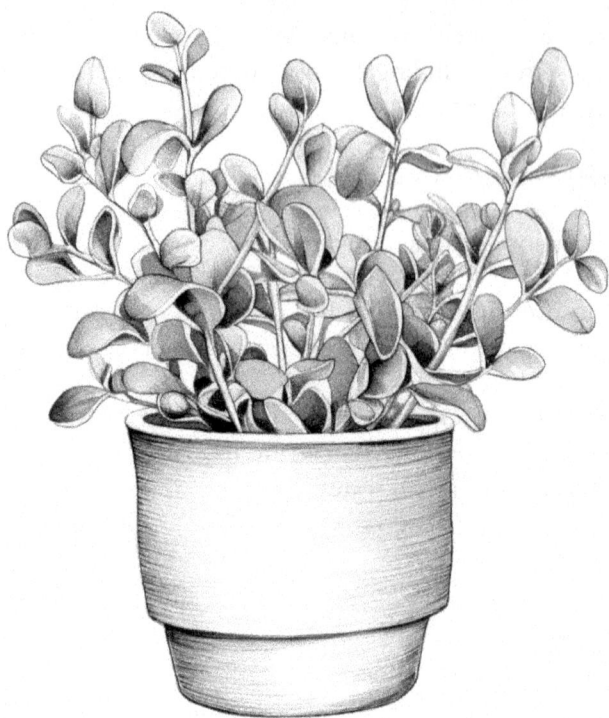

Eucalyptus

- **Healing applications**: This herb clears congestion and aids in breathing, fights bacterial infections, reduces inflammation in conditions like arthritis, soothes coughs and throat irritation, combats viral infections, eases symptoms of sinus infections, has antiseptic properties for wound care, invigorates the mind and improves focus, lowers fever associated with infections, alleviates muscle and joint pain, acts as a natural insect deterrent, enhances the immune system, aids in relaxation and stress relief, supports oral health, and is used for its soothing aroma in aromatherapy.

- **Side effects**: skin irritation, nausea, or vomiting

- **Native habitat**: Native to Australia, this herb can also be found in California, Florida, Texas, Arizona, and other American states.

- **Part(s) used**: leaves and oil

- **Preparation**: essential oils, lozenges, teas, and chest rubs

- **Recommended dosage**: Do not take eucalyptus oil internally. Inhale the vapor instead. For tea, use eucalyptus leaves—1 to 1.5 teaspoons per cup of tea.

- **Application methods**: Inhale the oil vapor, brew it into tea, or topically apply a dilute version of the oil.

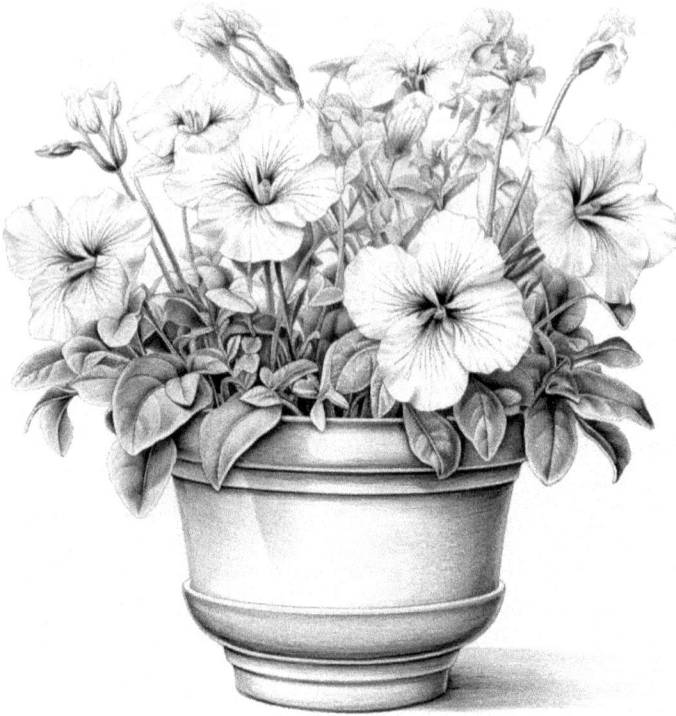

Evening Primrose

- **Healing applications**: supports women's health during menstruation and menopause, alleviates eczema and dermatitis symptoms, reduces inflammation in conditions like arthritis, eases symptoms of rheumatoid arthritis, supports heart health and reduces cholesterol, aids in managing nerve-related conditions, alleviates symptoms of diabetic neuropathy, helps in managing symptoms of asthma, eases symptoms of irritable bowel syndrome, supports bone density and reduces osteoporosis risk, may aid in symptom management, reduces symptoms of cyclic mastalgia, supports growth and health, may assist in weight loss efforts, and helps in managing allergy symptoms.

- **Side effects**: diarrhea and bleeding

- **Native habitat**: It originated in North America and grows in states like California, Texas, New York, Ohio, and others.

- **Part(s) used**: leaves seeds and roots

- **Preparation**: capsules, oil extracts, and creams

- **Recommended dosage**: 500 to 1,500 mg of oil daily

- **Application methods**: Apply creams topically and take capsules and powders orally.

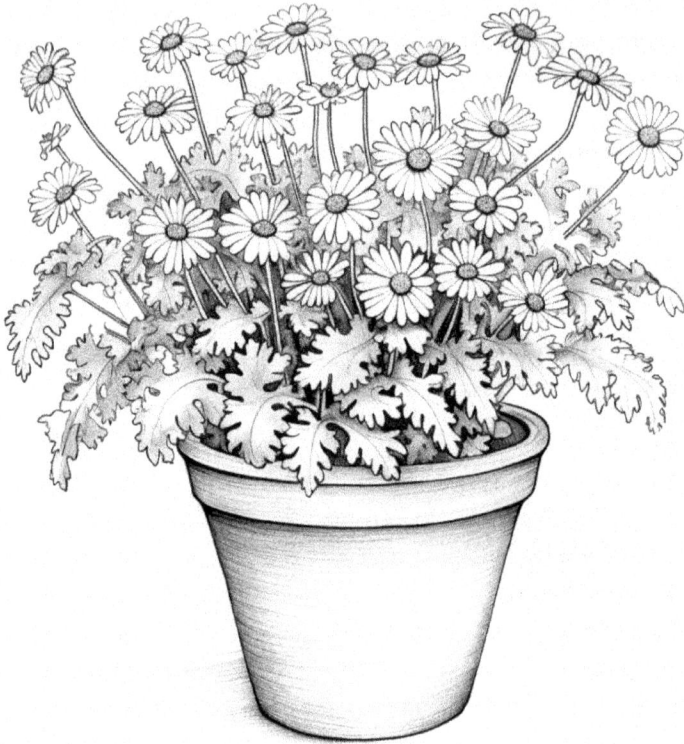

Feverfew

- **Healing applications**: The herb reduces the frequency and severity of migraines, alleviates symptoms of rheumatoid arthritis, lowers fever associated with infections, eases symptoms of indigestion and bloating, relieves symptoms like cramps and discomfort, mitigates symptoms of hay fever, reduces inflammation in joints, treats dermatitis and psoriasis symptoms, eases tension headaches, reduces symptoms related to nausea, aids in managing symptoms of dizziness, alleviates symptoms of various rheumatic conditions, helps in managing symptoms, eases symptoms of colitis and irritable bowel syndrome, and acts as a mild sedative.

- **Side effects**: High doses may cause mouth ulcers or gastrointestinal upset.

- **Native habitat**: It is native to Europe and Asia but also grows in many U.S. states such as New York, California, Texas, Florida, and others.

- **Part(s) used**: leaves and flowers

- **Preparation**: powders, tablets, tinctures, and teas

- **Recommended dosage**: 50–100 mg of dried leaves or its equivalent for powders, tinctures, and teas.

- **Application methods**: Take this herb in tea, hot water, or a beverage.

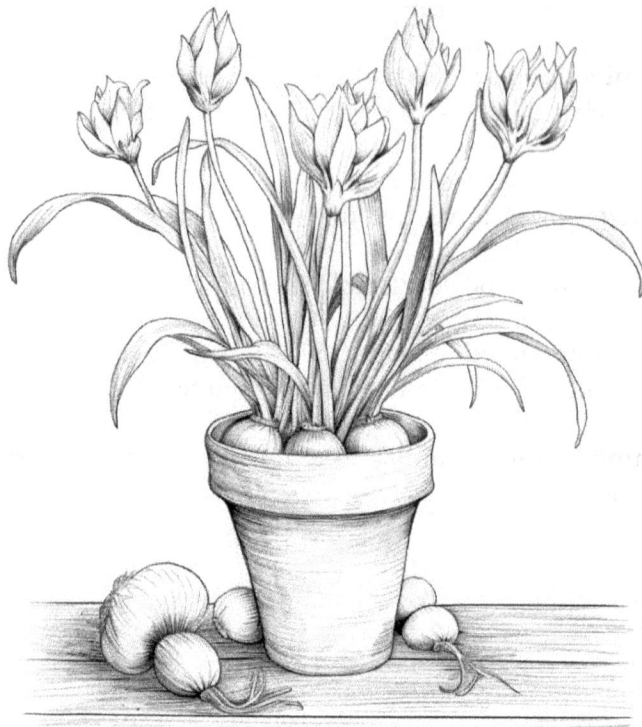

Garlic

- **Healing applications**: The herb lowers blood pressure and cholesterol, fights infections, including respiratory issues, boosts the immune system, reduces inflammation in arthritis, exhibits potential anti-cancer properties, protects against oxidative stress, combats fungal infections, aids in diabetes management, relieves indigestion and bloating, acts as a natural immune booster, may reduce allergy symptoms, has antiseptic properties, eases symptoms of osteoarthritis, supports liver function, and is traditionally used for enhancing libido.

- **Side effects**: Some people may experience stomach upset or skin rashes, especially with high doses.

- **Native habitat**: Native to Central Asia, this plant also grows in California, Texas, New York, and Oregon.

- **Part(s) used**: bulbs

- **Preparation**: fresh cloves, garlic oil, powder, capsules, and pure extracts of aged garlic

- **Recommended dosage**: 600 to 1200 mg of purified extract or 2–4 garlic cloves daily

- **Application methods**: You can eat garlic raw or cook it in food.

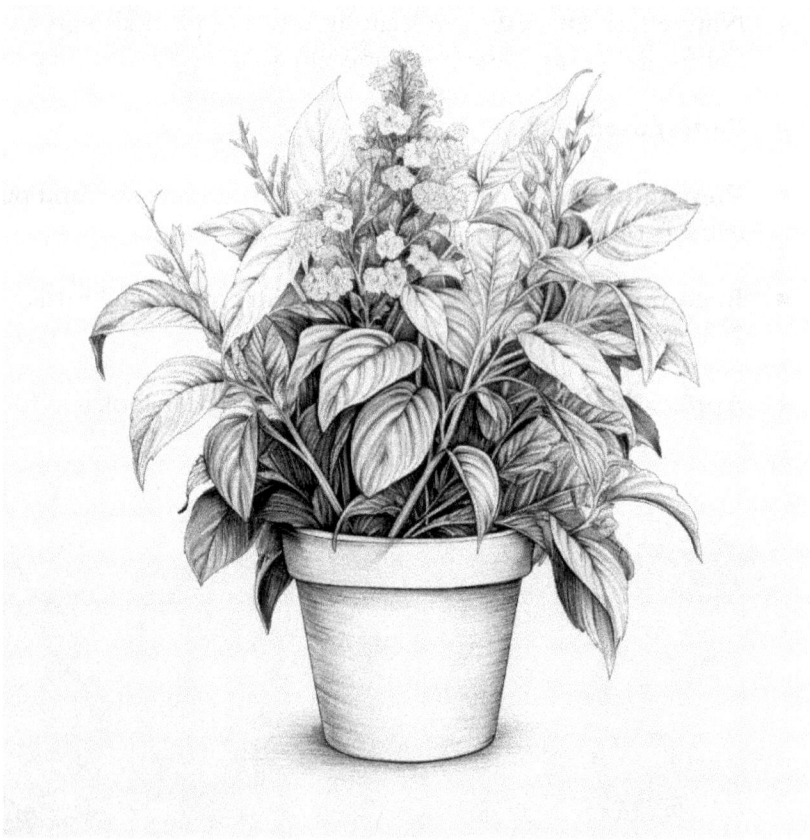

Ginger

- **Healing applications**: It relieves nausea, indigestion, and bloating, reduces inflammation in arthritis, eases symptoms of morning sickness and motion sickness, alleviates migraine headaches, reduces cramps and discomfort, relieves symptoms of colds and respiratory infections, exhibits potential anti-cancer properties, aids in diabetes management, eases symptoms of osteoarthritis, lowers blood pressure and cholesterol, fights bacterial infections, supports weight loss efforts, assists in managing nausea during chemotherapy, has calming effects on the nervous system, and alleviates muscle soreness and pain.

- **Side effects**: may cause heartburn or bleeding if taken in high doses

- **Native habitat**: It's native to Southeast Asia and also available in Texas, Florida, California, Hawaii, and other states.

- **Part(s) used**: rhizomes

- **Preparation**: fresh ginger, tea, powders, oils, and extracts

- **Recommended dosage**: 1–2 grams of ginger daily

- **Application methods**: You can consume ginger fresh as a juice, in tea, or cooked in foods.

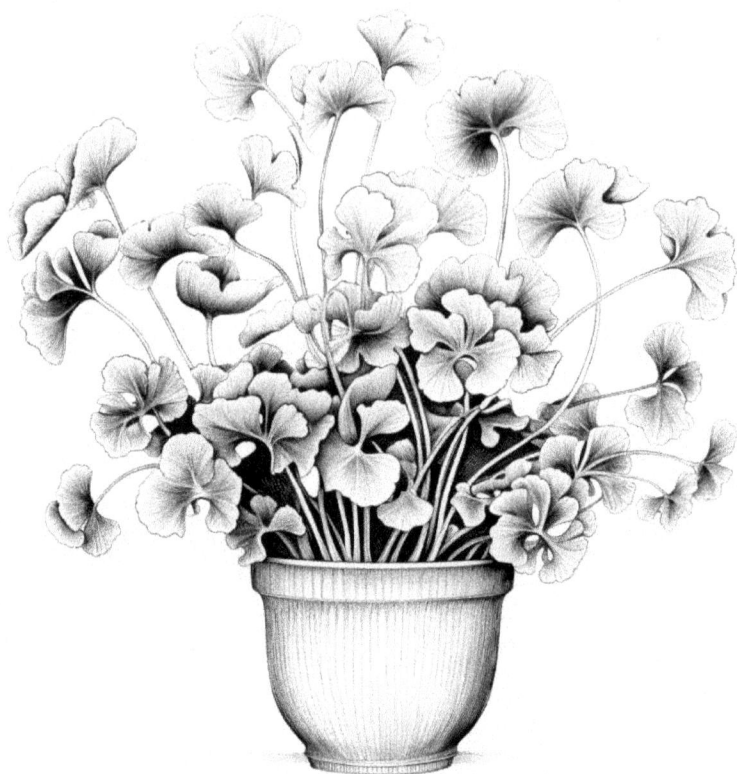

Ginkgo Biloba

- **Healing applications**: It improves memory and cognitive performance, combats oxidative stress, enhances blood flow in extremities, supports eye health, may alleviate glaucoma symptoms, reduces the frequency and severity of migraines, may alleviate symptoms, improves symptoms of ringing in the ears, aids in recovery post-stroke, helps control asthma symptoms, alleviates symptoms of this circulatory disorder, may aid in symptom management, reduces inflammation in various conditions, assists in managing blood sugar levels, improves symptoms in men and women, and has the potential for mitigating cognitive effects.

- **Side effects**: may cause stomach upset or skin rash

- **Native habitat**: Native to China, this herb can also be found in California, Texas, Florida, New York, and other U.S. locations.

- **Part(s) used**: leaves

- **Preparation**: powders, tinctures, and tea

- **Recommended dosage**: 120 to 240 mg

- **Application methods**: You can brew it into tea or mix the tincture with your beverages.

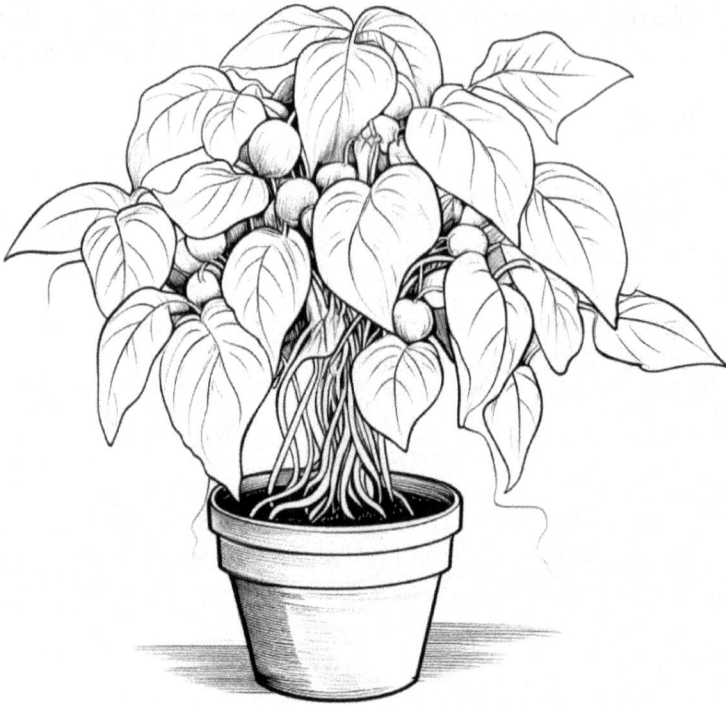

Ginseng

- **Healing applications**: This plant increases stamina and reduces fatigue, helps the body adapt to stress, improves memory and mental clarity, strengthens the immune system, regulates blood sugar levels, combats oxidative stress, supports heart health, reduces inflammation in arthritis, exhibits potential anti-cancer properties, aids in erectile dysfunction and libido, alleviates symptoms of asthma, acts as a mild antidepressant, relieves hot flashes and mood swings, assists in weight loss efforts, and enhances physical performance.

- **Side effects**: insomnia or stomach upset

- **Native habitat**: It is native to North America and grows in many states including Georgia, Pennsylvania, Wisconsin, and North Carolina.

- **Part(s) used**: roots

- **Preparation**: powders, refined extracts, and dried root

- **Recommended dosage**: 200–400 mg of refined extracts or 1–2 grams of dried roots

- **Application methods**: Use the dried or fresh roots of this herb to brew tea or make tinctures for use in beverages. It's also available in the form of energy drinks.

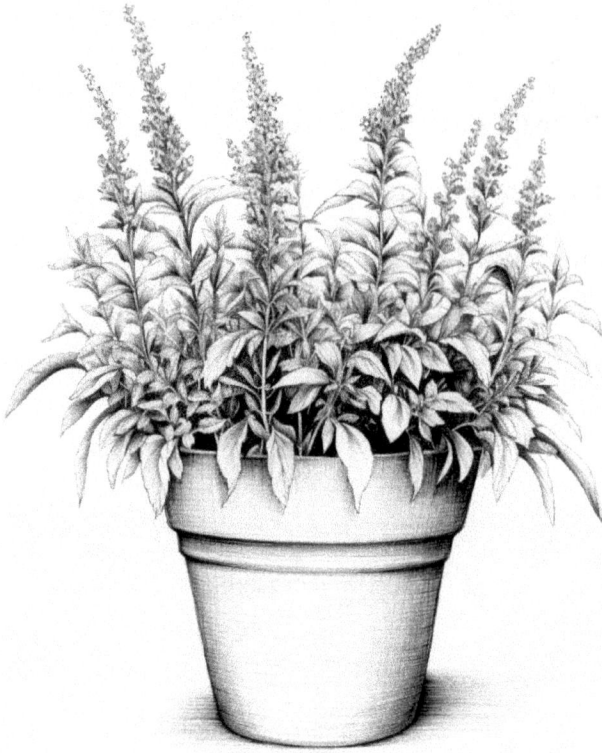

Goldenrod

- **Healing applications**: The herb treats urinary infections and kidney stones, eases joint pain and arthritis, relieves symptoms of bronchitis and asthma, supports wound and burn recovery, alleviates indigestion and gastrointestinal issues, manages symptoms of hay fever and allergies, supports liver function, combats fungal infections, fights bacterial infections, improves blood circulation, treats eczema and dermatitis, relieves muscle spasms, lowers fever associated with infections, has calming effects on the nervous system, and assists in managing blood sugar levels.

- **Side effects**: skin irritation, stomach upset, gastrointestinal issues

- **Native habitat**: It originated in North America and grows in many states, such as New York, California, Texas, Florida, and more.

- **Part(s) used**: leaves and flowers

- **Preparation**: tinctures, teas, capsules, and creams

- **Recommended dosage**: 1 to 2 teaspoons or 2 to 4 milliliters of tincture thrice daily

- **Application methods**: Use the dry leaves and flowers to brew tea or steep in hot water. You can also add the tincture to your beverages.

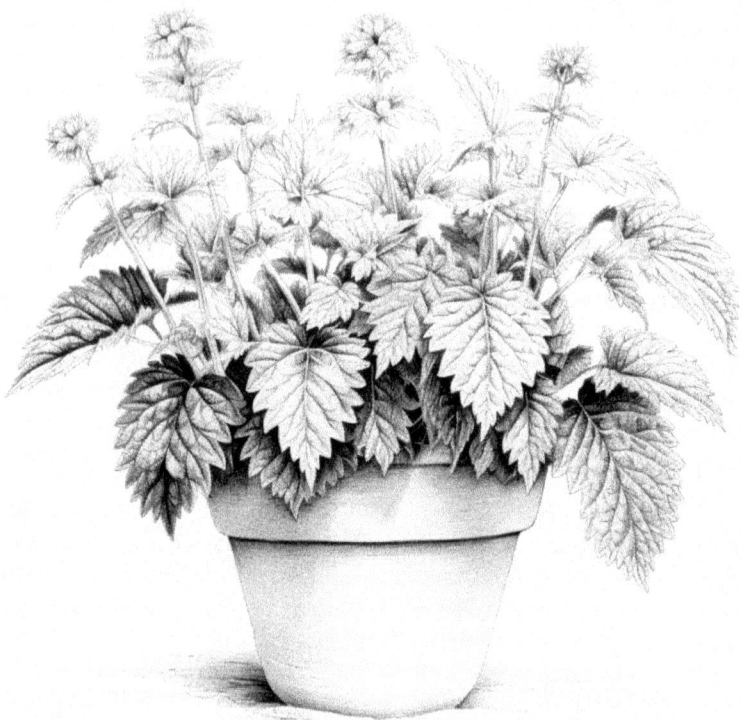

Goldenseal

- **Healing applications**: It's an herb that boosts the immune system, alleviates indigestion and promotes digestion, fights bacterial infections, combats viral infections, reduces inflammation in various conditions, eases symptoms of colds and respiratory infections, treats eczema, rashes, and wounds, manages conjunctivitis and other eye infections, supports kidney and bladder health, aids in managing diarrhea, promotes gum health and alleviates mouth sores, relieves symptoms like cramps, exhibits potential anti-cancer properties, manages allergy symptoms, and supports liver function.

- **Side effects**: Stomach upset and elevated blood pressure are some potential allergies.

- **Native habitat**: Native to North America, you can find it in states like Kentucky, Ohio, West Virginia, Georgia, and others.

- **Part(s) used**: rhizomes and roots

- **Preparation**: powders, tinctures, powders, and ointments

- **Recommended dosage**: 500–2000 mg of root powder or 30–120 tincture drops daily

- **Application methods**: You can take this herb in beverages, brew it into tea, or steep it in hot water. Apply the ointment externally for eczema.

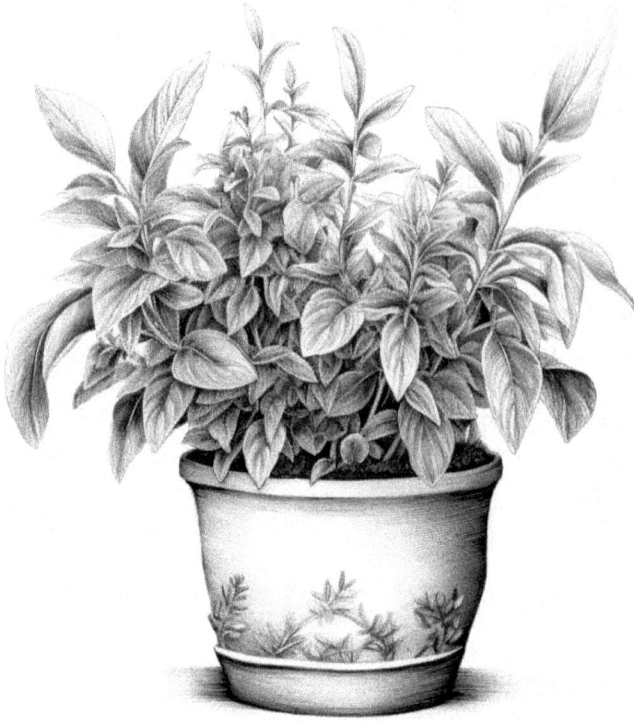

Green Tea

- **Healing applications**: It combats oxidative stress, reduces cholesterol and lowers blood pressure, supports weight loss efforts, exhibits potential anti-cancer properties, improves cognitive function and reduces the risk of Alzheimer's, reduces inflammation in various conditions, regulates blood sugar levels, supports liver function, prevents cavities and improves oral hygiene, treats acne and promotes skin health, fights bacterial infections, improves symptoms of asthma and bronchitis, delays signs of aging due to rich antioxidants, has a calming effect on the nervous system, and alleviates symptoms like cramps.

- **Side effects**: Some potential adverse reactions to this herb are jitteriness, insomnia, or digestive issues when you take high doses.

- **Native habitat**: Native to East Asia, it also grows in states like Hawaii, California, Oregon, Washington, and more.

- **Part(s) used**: leaves and leaf buds.

- **Preparation**: loose leaves, tea bags, extracts, and supplements

- **Recommended dosage**: 1 to 3 cups of tea or 100 to 750 mg of powder daily

- **Application methods**: You can take this herb in beverages, brew it into tea, or steep it in hot water. Apply the ointment externally.

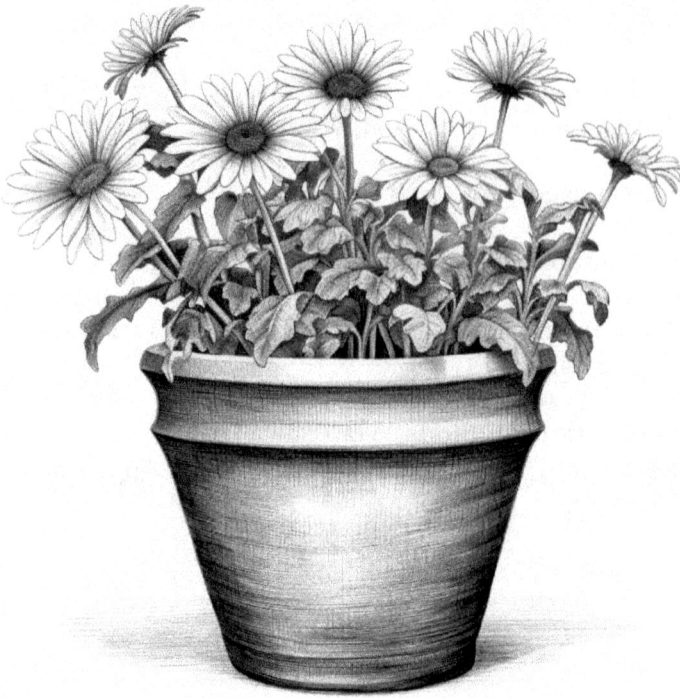

Grindelia

- **Healing applications**: It is used to treat asthma, bronchitis, persistent cough, arthritis, eczema, dermatitis, mucus, muscle spasms, urinary infections, bacterial infections, wounds, indigestion, nervous tension, and insomnia. It also improves heart health and fluid balance.

- **Side effects**: It may cause stomach upset, rashes, and nausea.

- **Native habitat**: This plant can be found in California, Oregon, Washington, Arizona, Nevada, New Mexico, Colorado, Utah, and Texas.

- **Part(s) used**: leaves, flowers, and stems

- **Preparation**: tinctures, teas, capsules, and a liquid extract

- **Recommended dosage**: 1–4 grams or 2–4 mL of tincture daily (three times)

- **Application methods**: You can take this herb in tea or as capsules and tinctures.

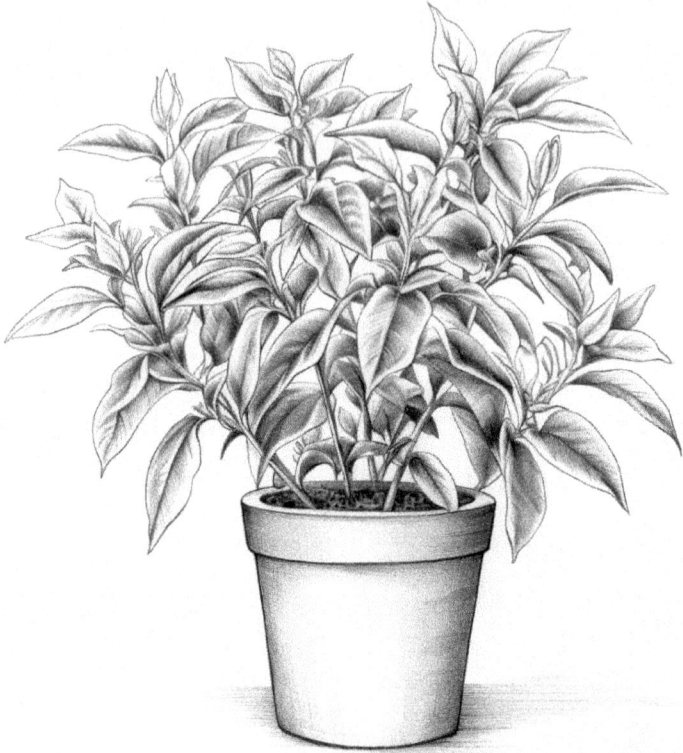

Guarana

- **Healing applications**: The seeds of this herb contain a high
  amount of caffeine. Use this herb to increase mental focus and
  clarity, alertness and stamina, and urine flow. It is also great for
  suppressing appetite, oxidative stress, and discomfort. It is also
  effective against migraine, indigestion, heart diseases, premature
  aging, moodiness, inflammation, and respiratory conditions.
  People can use it to enhance libido and lower body temperature.

- **Side effects**: insomnia and overstimulation of the nervous
  system due to the caffeine content.

- **Native habitat**: Its origin can be traced back to Brazil, but it grows in many American states, such as Hawaii, Puerto Rico, and Florida.

- **Part(s) used**: seeds

- **Preparation**: powders, capsules, tinctures, and energy drinks.

- **Recommended dosage**: 100–200 mg daily (22% caffeine)

- **Application methods**: taken as capsules, energy drinks, or in beverages

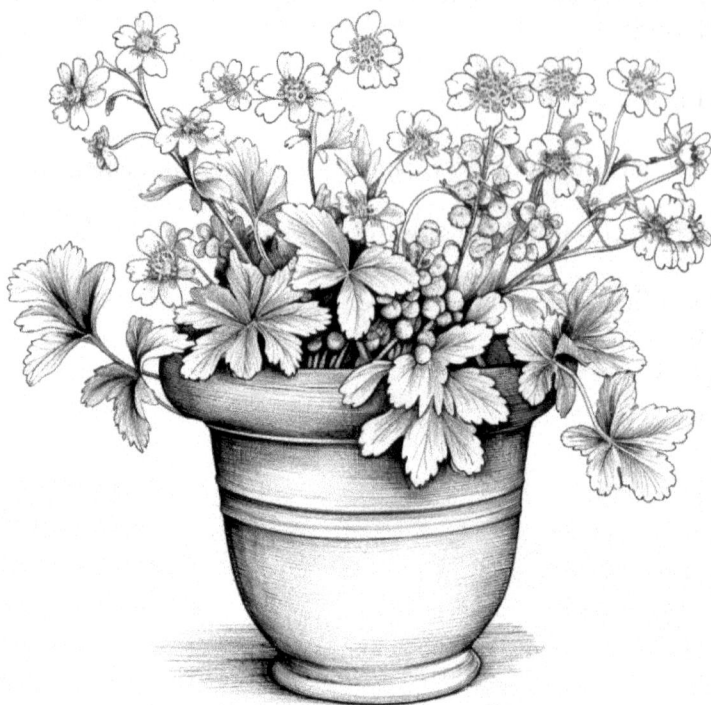

Hawthorn

- **Healing applications**: Use it to manage hypertension, heart problems, indigestion, nervous tension, oxidative stress, lower cholesterol, enhance immune function, treat insomnia, alleviate discomfort, improve urine flow, lose weight, and relax.

- **Side effects**: Stomach cramps, nausea, and headaches are some possible adverse reactions.

- **Native habitat**: This plant grows in several American states, including California, Texas, Florida, New York, Illinois, Ohio, Michigan, and Pennsylvania.

- **Part(s) used**: leaves, berries, and flowers

- **Preparation**: teas, tinctures, and capsules

- **Recommended dosage**: 160–1,800 mg daily

- **Application methods**: Take it in tea or orally as capsules and tinctures.

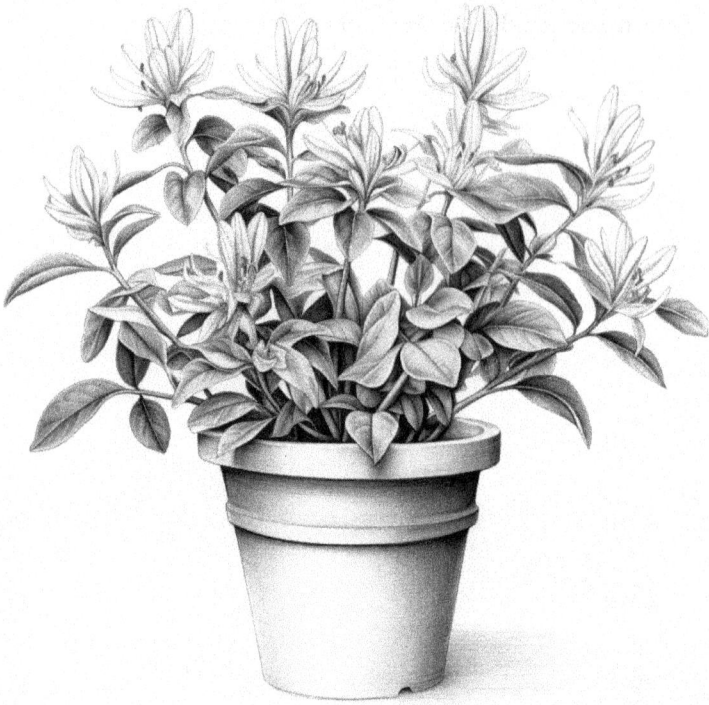

Honeysuckle

- **Healing applications**: It reduces inflammation, oxidative stress, and body temperature; alleviates cough, asthma, and indigestion; and treats rashes, eczema, liver problems, headaches, and joint pain. It prevents cancer and nervous tension, manages cholesterol, and strengthens the immune system.

- **Side effects**: Diarrhea, nausea, itching, and redness are some potential adverse reactions.

- **Native habitat**: Some American states where you can find this plant are Missouri, Tennessee, Texas, California, Florida, New York, Georgia, Virginia, Ohio, Illinois, North Carolina, and Pennsylvania.

- **Part(s) used**: flowers, leaves, and stems

- **Preparation**: teas, tinctures, extracts, and capsules

- **Recommended dosage**: 2–15 grams of powder or 4.5–30 mL of tincture

- **Application methods**: You can consume this herb in tea, beverages, and food, or take it in the form of capsules.

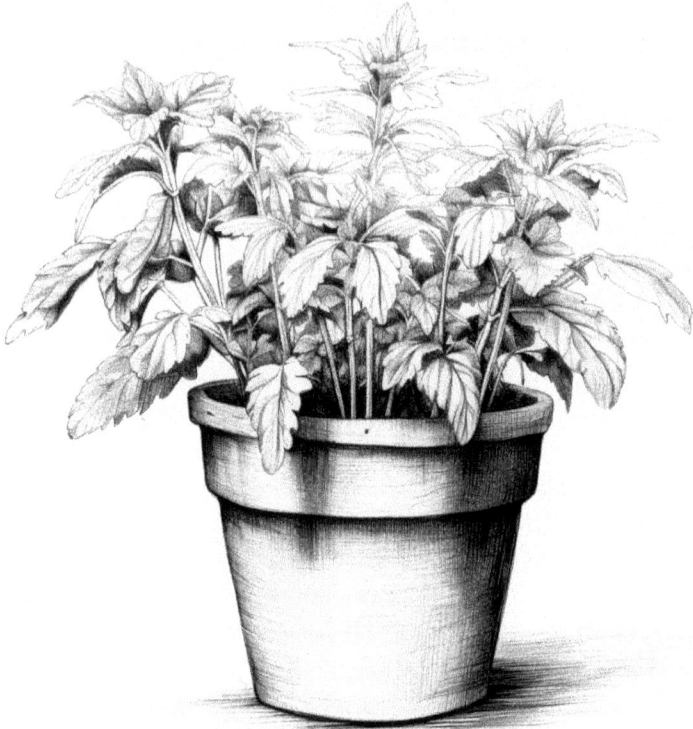

Horseradish

- **Healing applications:** This plant is used to relieve nasal congestion, indigestion, and inflammation, prevent infections, improve blood flow, support the liver, and alleviate stress. It can also relieve joint pain, headaches, and muscle pain, inhibit bacterial growth, and enhance immune function.

- **Side effects:** Some known adverse reactions are skin redness, irritation, and stomach upset.

- **Native habitat:** It is native to Europe but also grows in Illinois, Wisconsin, Michigan, Ohio, Indiana, Pennsylvania, New York, California, Oregon, Washington, Texas, and Florida.

- **Part(s) used:** roots

- **Preparation:** tinctures, extracts, and capsules

- **Recommended dosage:** 1–2 teaspoons of powder daily

- **Application methods:** You can eat it raw, add it to dishes, or consume it as tinctures or teas.

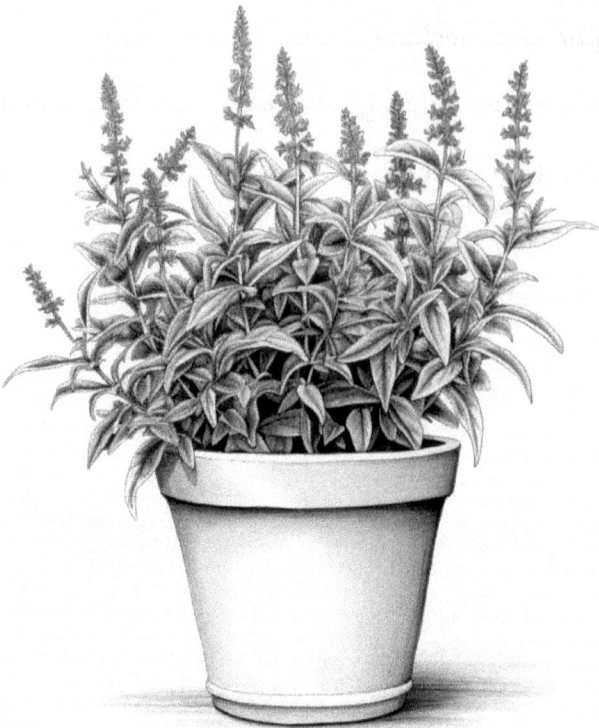

Hyssop

- **Healing applications**: Use this herb to relieve coughs, nasal congestion, inflammation, oxidative stress, and nervous tension. It can also fight viral, bacterial, and parasitic infections. Use it for skin conditions, indigestion, better blood flow, cramps, urine flow, and improving the immune system.

- **Side effects**: Itching, skin rashes, nausea, and diarrhea are all potential allergies.

- **Native habitat**: Originating from Mediterranean countries, this plant also grows in California, Oregon, Washington, Texas, New York, Pennsylvania, Virginia, North Carolina, Georgia, Ohio, Michigan, and Colorado.

- **Part(s) used**: leaves and flowers

- **Preparation**: teas, tinctures, essential oils, and capsules

- **Recommended dosage**: 1–4 grams of powder or 2–4 mL of tincture thrice a day

- **Application methods**: Make delicious teas from this herb or use the tinctures and oils in beverages. You can also take it in capsule form.

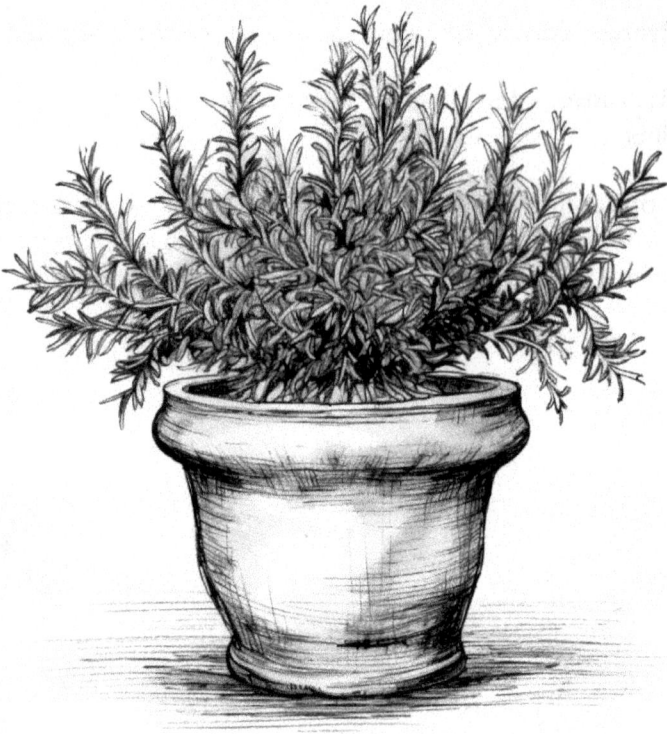

Juniper

- **Healing applications**: It treats or relieves infections, indigestion, inflammation, nasal congestion, oxidative stress, arthritis, bacterial infections, cramps, parasitic infections, eczema, psoriasis, and rheumatism. It also aids urine flow, blood flow, and liver health.

- **Side effects**: Itching, redness, upset stomach, and nausea are some adverse reactions associated with this herb.

- **Native habitat**: It grows worldwide, and you can find it in states like Wyoming, Montana, Idaho, Nevada, California Texas, Arizona, Colorado, Utah, Oregon, Washington, and New Mexico.

- **Part(s) used**: berries and leaves

- **Preparation**: teas, tinctures, essential oils, and capsules

- **Recommended dosage**: 2–10 grams of crushed berries or 1 to 4 mL of tinctures

- **Application methods**: It is usually taken orally as tea or added to beverages such as tinctures and essential oils.

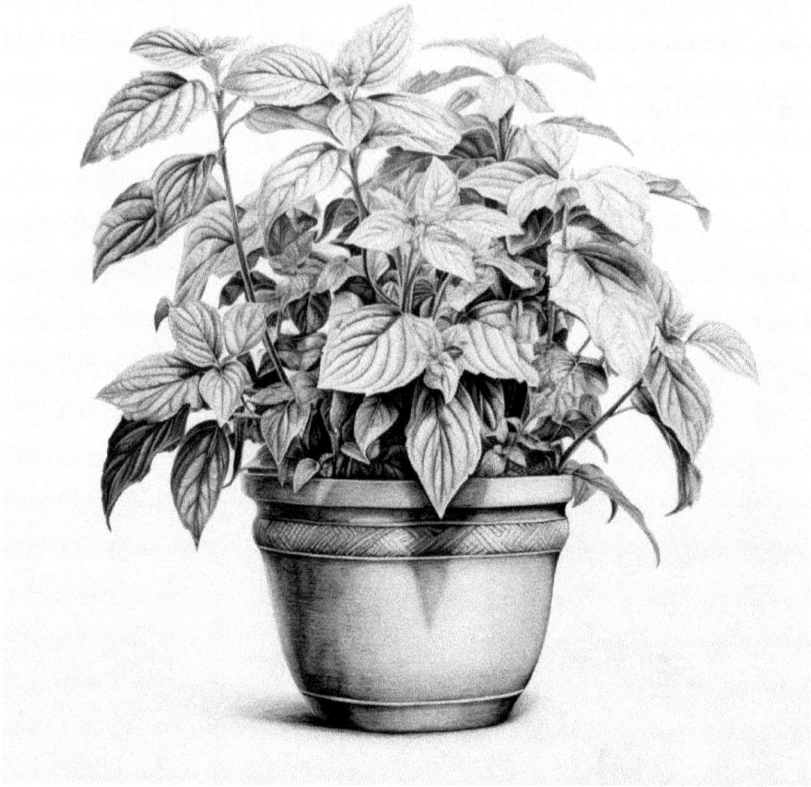

Kava Kava

- **Healing applications**: It reduces anxiety, tension, depression, and oxidative stress. It is a good remedy for mental confusion, pains, inflammation, muscle spasms, infections, cramps, asthma, and cancer. This herb can also improve liver health and your mood.

- **Side effects**: Excesses may cause liver toxicity and skin rashes.

- **Native habitat**: It is native to the South Pacific and also does well in states like Hawaii, Florida, California, Texas, Louisiana, Puerto Rico, Georgia, South Carolina, Alabama, Mississippi, Arizona, and New Mexico.

- **Part(s) used**: roots

- **Preparation**: teas, tinctures, capsules, and extracts

- **Recommended dosage**: 60 to 300 mg of powder daily

- **Application methods**: Use this herb to brew tea or make tinctures that can be added to beverages and food.

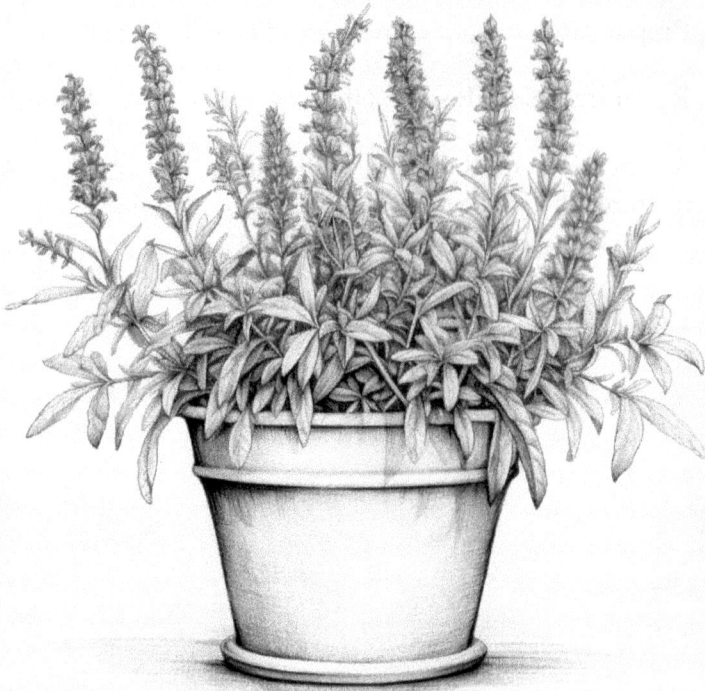

Lavender

- **Healing applications**: People use this herb to treat anxiety, insomnia, restlessness, migraines, headaches, inflammation, dermatitis, wounds, burns, infections, coughs, congestion, indigestion, nausea, disinfect cuts, improve mood, and ease tension. It is also effective against muscle cramps and fungal infections, and it's a good agent for boosting memory and keeping insects away.

- **Side effects**: Some adverse reactions include itching, rashes, and disrupted hormone levels.

- **Native habitat**: Lavender is native to Mediterranean countries but grows in California, Texas, Oregon, Washington, New York,

Michigan, Virginia, North Carolina, Georgia, Colorado, New Mexico, and Arizona.

- **Part(s) used**: flowers, leaves, and essential oils

- **Preparation**: essential oils, teas, tinctures, and capsules

- **Recommended dosage**: 80–160 mg of essential oil daily

- **Application methods**: Take this herb as a tea or use its tinctures and oils in foods and beverages.

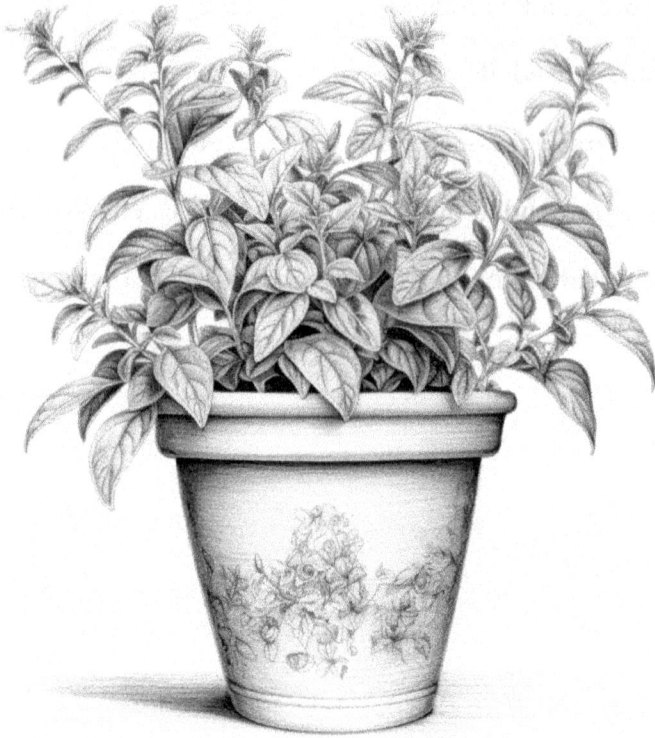

Lemon Balm

- **Healing applications**: This herb has many uses, including, anxiety relief, promoting relaxation for better sleep, cognitive function, antiviral properties, digestive aid, anti-inflammatory agent, mood enhancement, speeding up healing, headache relief, respiratory health, menstrual pain, antioxidant support, thyroid health, immune boosting, and fighting the herpes simplex virus.

- **Side effects**: Some individuals may experience drowsiness, skin irritation, or rash

- **Native habitat**: Native to the Mediterranean region, this plant grows in California, Texas, Florida, New York, Illinois, Ohio,

Pennsylvania, Virginia, North Carolina, Georgia, Michigan, and Oregon.

- **Part(s) used**: leaves and flowers

- **Preparation**: teas, tinctures, capsules, and essential oils

- **Recommended dosage**: 300 to 1,500 mg daily

- **Application methods**: You can brew tea, add tincture to your drink, integrate it into your recipes, or swallow capsule pills.

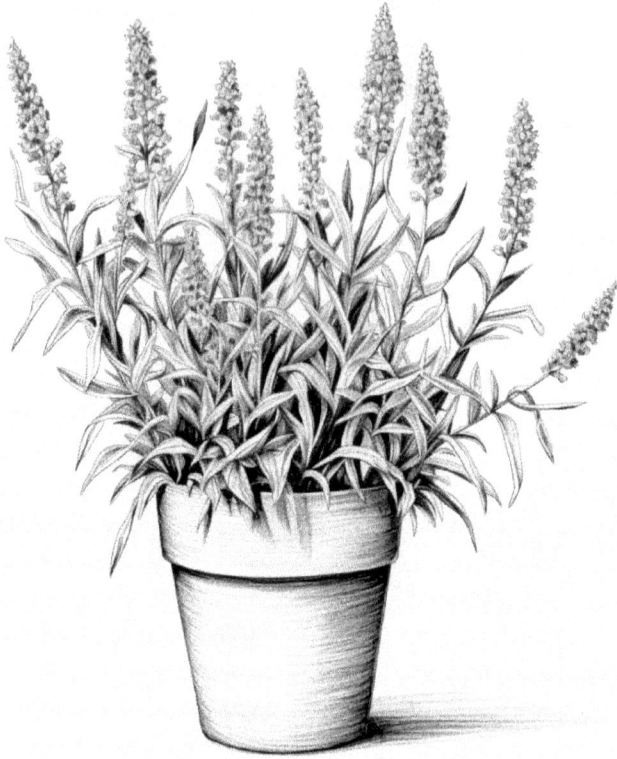

Licorice Root

- **Healing applications**: This herb performs the following functions: relieves coughs and bronchitis, treats indigestion and ulcers, balances stress hormones, reduces inflammation, boosts immune function, relieves PMS symptoms, destroys viruses, aids liver function, alleviates hot flashes, eases allergy symptoms, inhibits bacterial growth, treats psoriasis and eczema, improves memory, can aid weight loss, and soothes throat discomfort.

- **Side effects**: may elevate blood pressure and lower potassium levels

- **Native habitat**: It originated in Southern Europe but can grow in California, Texas, Arizona, New Mexico, Florida, Georgia, North Carolina, Virginia, Maryland, and Delaware.

- **Part(s) used**: roots and underground stems

- **Preparation**: teas, capsules, extracts, and powders.

- **Recommended dosage**: 250 to 500 mg daily

- **Application methods**: You can brew tea with it and use it in your meals and beverages. It's okay to take the powder directly or in hot water.

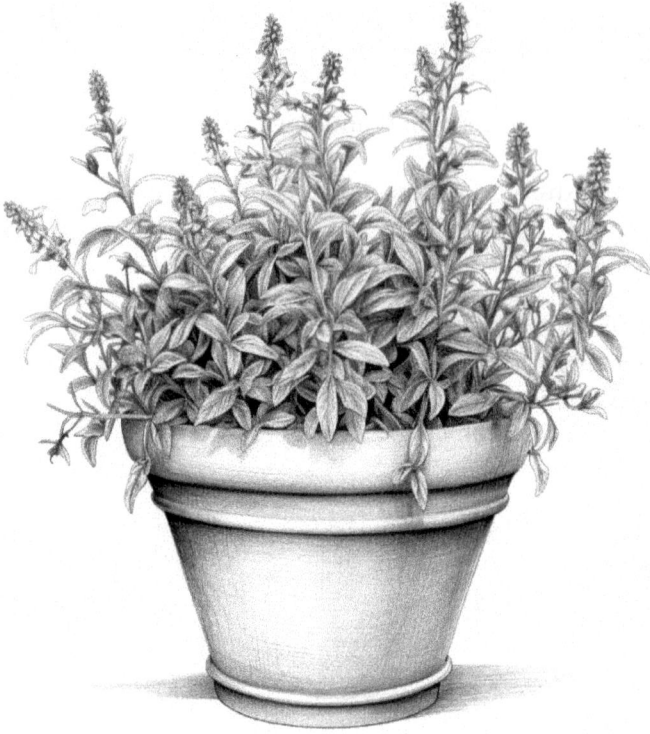

Lobelia

- **Healing applications**: It relieves asthma and bronchitis, eases muscle spasms, alleviates coughs, reduces inflammation, addresses indigestion, eases headaches and joint pain, supports liver health, manages high blood pressure, promotes mucus clearance, reduces anxiety, lowers body temperature, inhibits bacterial growth, promotes urine flow, addresses parasitic infections, and aids in quitting smoking.

- **Side effects**: Nausea, sweating, and vomiting may occur.

- **Native habitat**: It is available in California, Texas, Florida, New York, Illinois, Ohio, Michigan, Pennsylvania, Georgia, Virginia, North Carolina, Indiana, and other U.S. states.

- **Part(s) used**: leaves and flowers

- **Preparation**: tinctures, teas, capsules, and other extracts

- **Recommended dosage**: 0.3–1 gram powder daily

- **Application methods**: Make a juice with lobelia as one of the ingredients, brew tea with it, or consume it in your foods and other beverages.

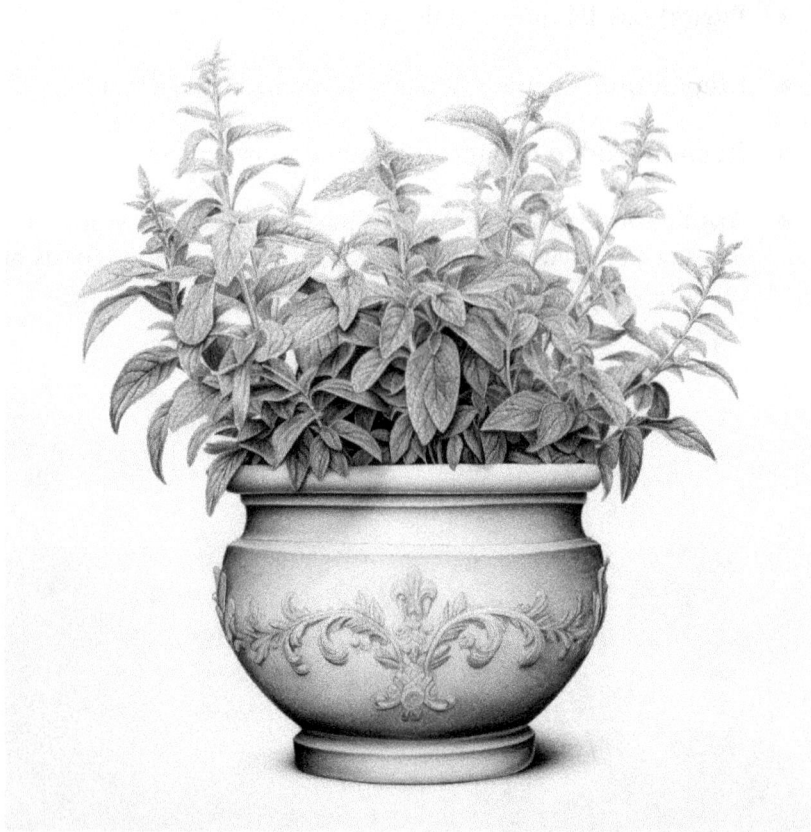

Ma Huang

- **Healing applications**: It relieves asthma and respiratory issues, alleviates nasal congestion, increases alertness and energy, acts as an appetite suppressant, reduces inflammation, alleviates allergy symptoms, enhances cognitive function, promotes urine flow, lowers body temperature, fights against viruses, manages low blood pressure, supports liver health, alleviates coughs, inhibits bacterial growth, and eases rheumatism symptoms.

- **Side effects**: may increase your heart rate or cause anxiety

- **Native habitat**: This plant is native to China and Mongolia but also grows in America in places like California, Nevada, Utah,

Arizona, New Mexico, Colorado, Wyoming, Montana, Idaho, Oregon, Washington, and Alaska.

- **Part(s) used**: dried stems

- **Preparation**: teas, capsules, extracts, and tinctures

- **Recommended dosage**: 6–30 mg daily

- **Application methods**: taken in tea, beverages, and swallowed as capsules

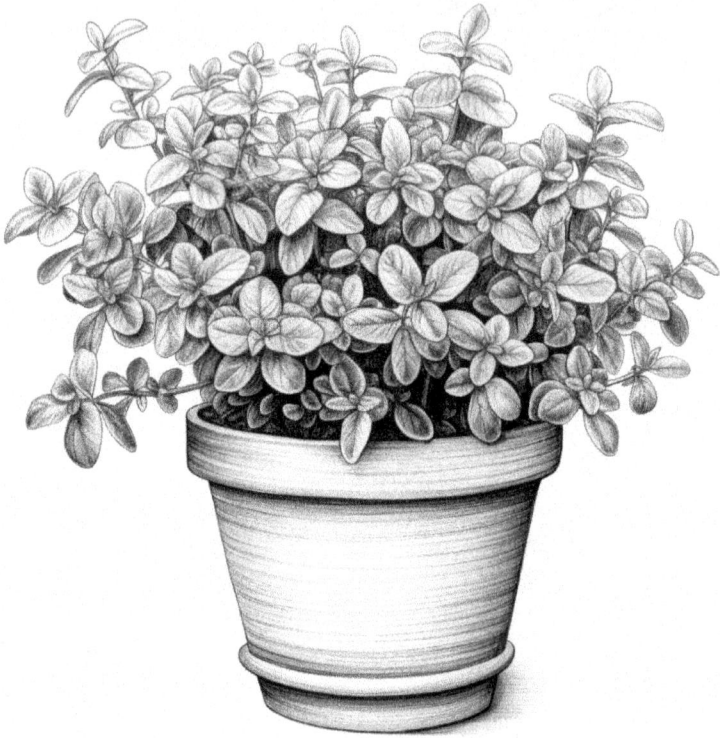

Marjoram

- **Healing applications**: This herb performs the following functions: eases indigestion, reduces inflammation, relieves coughs and congestion, eases headaches and muscle pain, combats oxidative stress, fights against infections, eases stress and anxiety, alleviates cramps, promotes relaxation for better sleep, supports digestion, enhances immune function, manages blood pressure, relieves muscle spasms, improves memory and focus, and treats skin irritations.

- **Side effects**: Potential adverse reactions include skin rash, itching, and low blood pressure.

- **Native habitat**: Native to the Mediterranean, this plant can also be found in California, Texas, Florida, New York, Illinois, Ohio, Pennsylvania, Virginia, North Carolina, Georgia, Michigan, and other states.

- **Part(s) used**: leaves and flowers

- **Preparation**: teas, essential oils, tinctures, and capsules

- **Recommended dosage**: 1–2 teaspoons of powder daily

- **Application methods**: You can brew tea with powder, leaves, or flowers. Some people take it in capsule form or add its essential oils to beverages and foods.

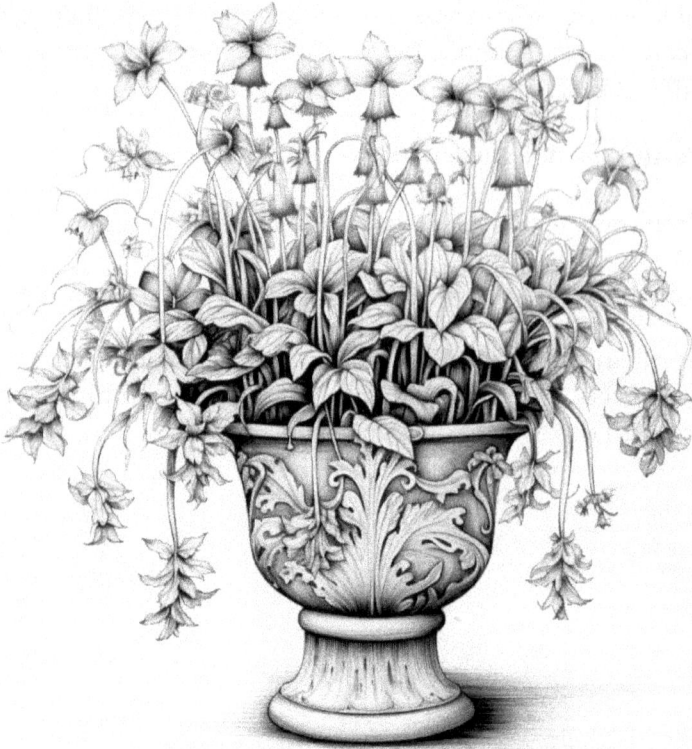

Marshmallow Root

- **Healing applications**: The herb has many uses. It relieves coughs and bronchitis, reduces inflammation, soothes indigestion and gastritis, alleviates infections, treats eczema and dermatitis, soothes throat discomfort, supports healing, inhibits bacterial growth, acts as a mild laxative, helps manage blood sugar levels, promotes skin recovery, eases arthritis discomfort, enhances immune function, addresses urinary issues, and alleviates persistent coughs.

- **Side effects**: rash, itching, low blood sugar

- **Native habitat**: It is native to Europe, Western Asia, and North Africa, but it also grows in California, Texas, Florida, New York,

Illinois, Ohio, Pennsylvania, Virginia, North Carolina, Georgia, Michigan, Missouri, and other states.

- **Part(s) used**: roots and leaves

- **Preparation**: teas, capsules, tinctures, and topical ointments

- **Recommended dosage**: 3–5 grams of dried roots or leaf extract

- **Application methods**: Make a delicious fruit beverage or juice with marshmallow root as an ingredient. You can also take the tincture directly or brew tea from the roots.

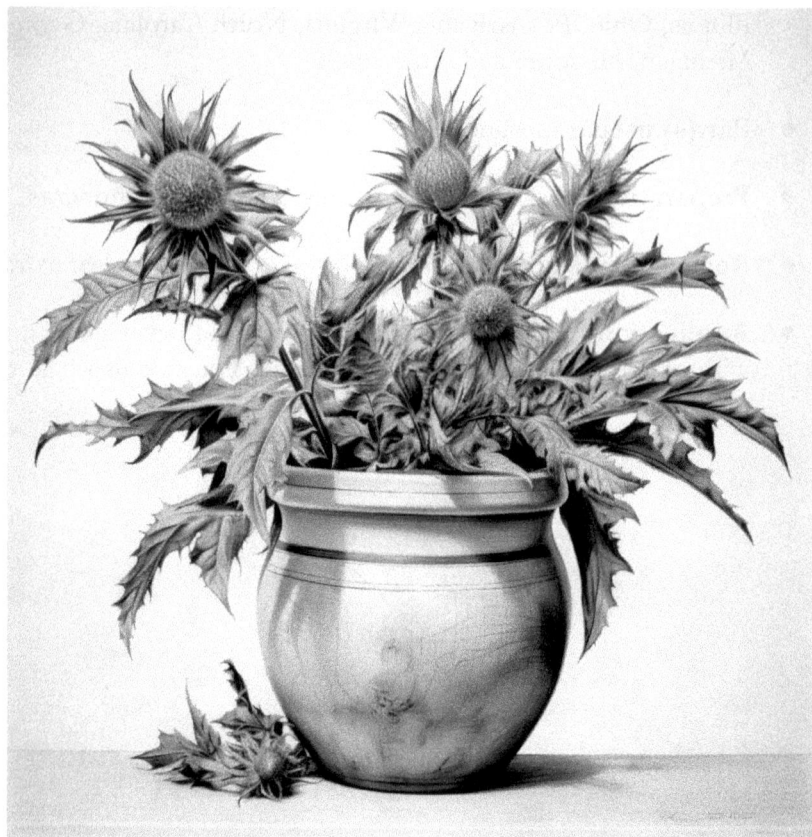

Milk Thistle

- **Healing applications**: It supports liver function, aids in detoxifying the liver, reduces inflammation, combats oxidative stress, supports gallbladder function, helps lower cholesterol levels, assists in managing blood sugar, eases indigestion and bloating, exhibits potential preventive effects, treats psoriasis, and acne, supports weight loss, manages blood pressure, supports kidney function, eases migraine symptoms, and increases bone strength.

- **Side effects**: Rash, itching, stomach upset, diarrhea, and nausea may occur.

- **Native habitat**: It originated from the Mediterranean region and grows in California, Texas, Florida, New York, Illinois, Ohio, Pennsylvania, Virginia, North Carolina, Georgia, Michigan, and Arizona.

- **Part(s) used**: seeds

- **Preparation**: powders, capsules, extracts, tinctures, and teas.

- **Recommended dosage**: 140–420 mg daily

- **Application methods**: You can swallow the capsules, but we recommend brewing tea with crushed or ground seeds or using its tinctures in beverages and other edibles.

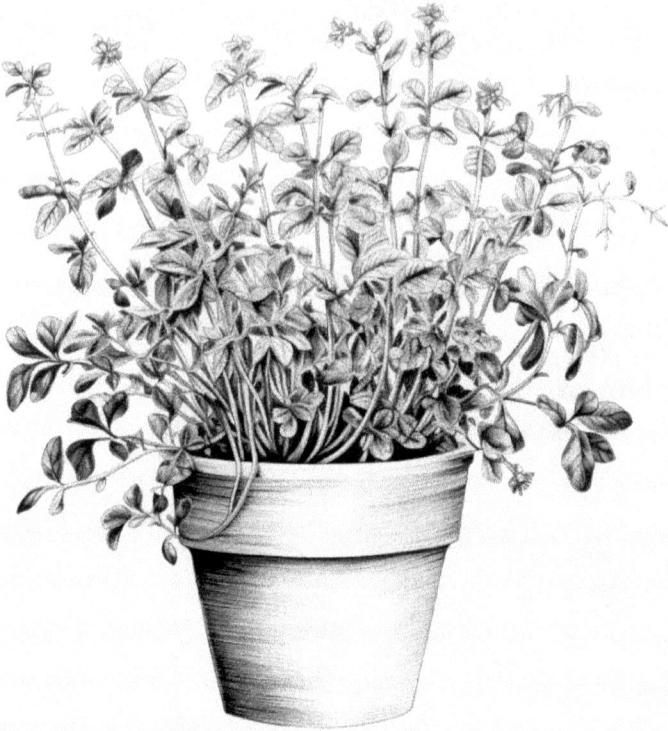

Moringa

- **Healing applications**: It's a superb source of essential vitamins and minerals, reduces inflammation, combats oxidative stress, helps manage diabetes, lowers cholesterol levels, inhibits bacterial growth, exhibits potential preventive effects, supports skin health, eases indigestion, aids in weight loss, enhances immune function, supports blood pressure control, eases arthritis symptoms, improves memory and focus, and alleviates allergy symptoms.

- **Side effects**: nausea, diarrhea, or low blood pressure if used excessively

- **Native habitat**: It is native to South Asia and now grows in Florida, Texas, California, Arizona, Hawaii, Puerto, Rico, Georgia, Louisiana, Mississippi, Alabama, South Carolina, North, and Carolina.

- **Part(s) used**: leaves, seeds, and pods

- **Preparation**: capsules, powders, teas, and other extracts

- **Recommended dosage**: 1.5 to 7 grams powder or 600–800 mg pure extract

- **Application methods**: You can ingest it directly, add it to a beverage, or brew tea with it.

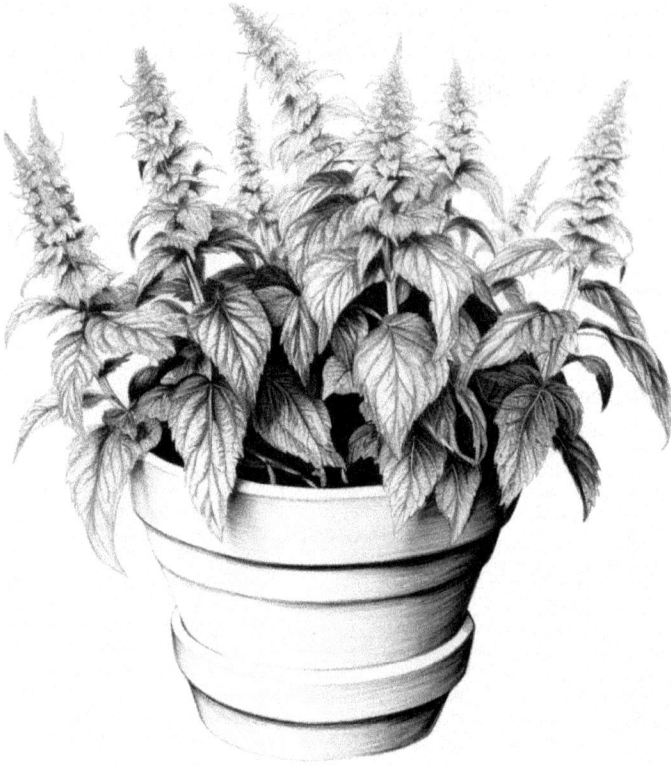

Motherwort

- **Healing applications**: The heart manages heart palpitations, eases menstrual cramps, calms nervous tension, supports uterine health, alleviates indigestion, reduces inflammation, relieves bronchitis symptoms, eases emotional stress, promotes relaxation for better sleep, balances thyroid function, inhibits bacterial growth, assists in recovery, supports liver function, promotes urine flow, and eases muscle spasms.

- **Side effects**: may cause nausea, diarrhea, or skin irritation

- **Native habitat**: Historically used in Europe, it grows in California, Texas, Florida, New York, Illinois, Ohio,

Pennsylvania, Virginia, North Carolina, Georgia, Michigan, Missouri, and many other states.

- **Part(s) used**: leaves and flowers

- **Preparation**: tinctures, teas, capsules, and other extracts

- **Recommended dosage**: 2 to 5 grams powder daily

- **Application methods**: You can brew tea from it, swallow the capsules, or add tinctures and other extracts to your food and beverages.

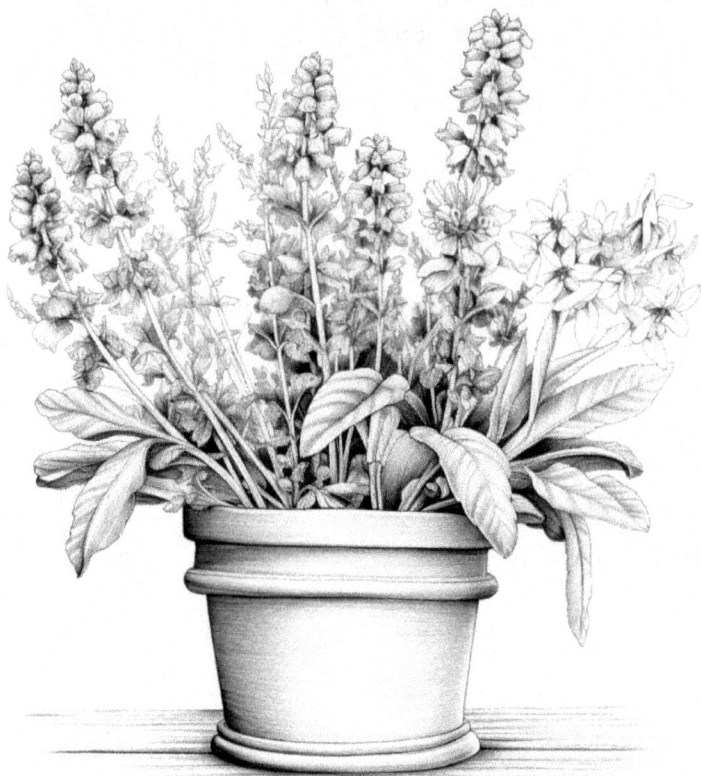

Mullein

- **Healing applications**: It relieves coughs and bronchitis, reduces inflammation, eases earache symptoms, promotes mucus clearance, eases arthritis discomfort, treats eczema and wounds, inhibits bacterial growth, promotes urine flow, fights against viruses, soothes indigestion, calms nervous tension, alleviates symptoms, relieves muscle spasms, manages blood pressure, and helps balance thyroid function.

- **Side effects**: skin irritation, itching, nausea, or diarrhea

- **Native habitat**: It is native to Europe, North Africa, and Asia. It grows in U.S. states like California, Texas, Florida, New York,

Illinois, Ohio, Pennsylvania, Virginia, North Carolina, Georgia, Michigan, Arizona, and more.

- **Part(s) used**: leaves and flowers

- **Preparation**: teas, tinctures, capsules, and other extracts

- **Recommended dosage**: 3 to 6 grams of ground leaves or flowers

- **Application methods**: Brew your tea with this herb or use it as a tincture in beverages and foods. You can also take the capsules.

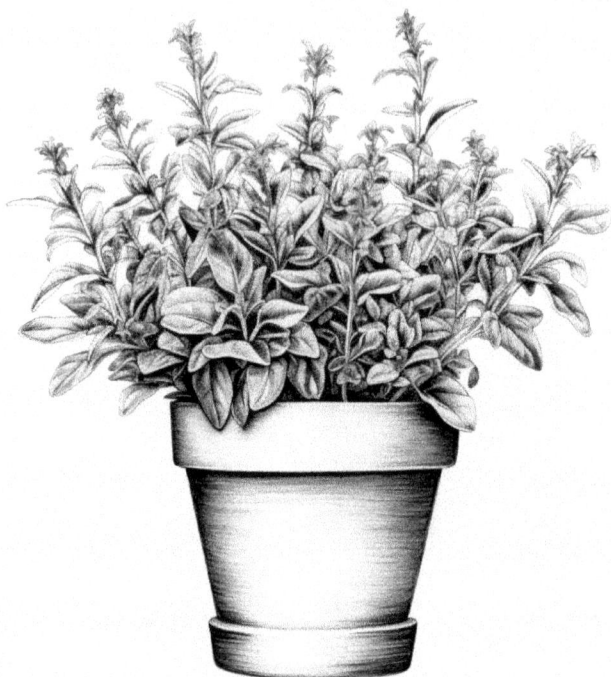

Mustard

- **Healing applications**: It relieves indigestion, eases congestion, reduces joint pain, alleviates soreness, supports liver health, manages cholesterol, inhibits bacterial growth, eases headaches, enhances blood flow, exhibits preventive effects, treats skin infections, boosts metabolism, treats dandruff, reduces inflammation, and induces relaxation.

- **Side effects**: skin redness, irritation, nausea, or abdominal

- **Native habitat**: You can find this herb in California, Kansas, North Dakota, South Dakota, Montana, Idaho, Oregon, Washington, Michigan, New York, and others.

- **Part(s) used**: seeds, leaves, and the oil

- **Preparation**: seeds, oil, poultices, and tinctures

- **Recommended dosage**: 1–2 teaspoons daily seeds or 1–2 tablespoons oil

- **Application methods**: You can take mustard with water, add the oil to your food, or apply the oil topically.

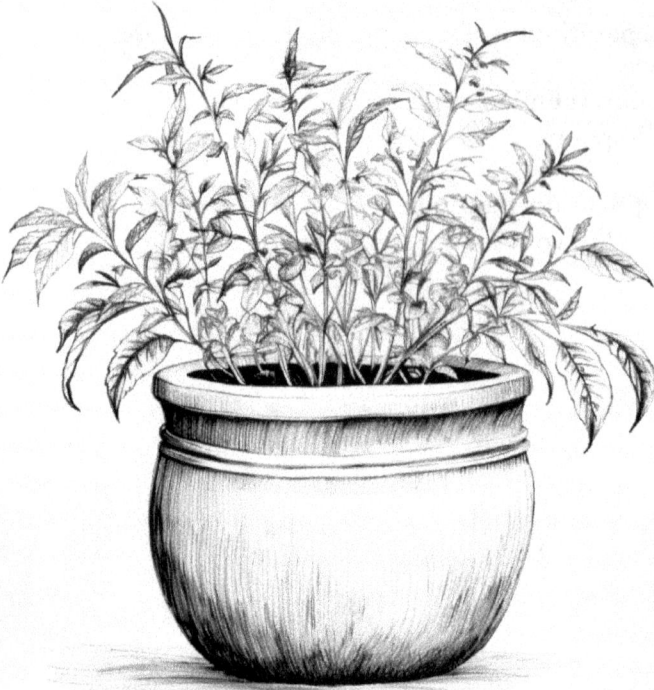

Neem

- **Healing applications**: Neem is used to treat acne, athlete's foot, various viral infections, arthritis, oxidative stress, eczema, and psoriasis, is used in toothpaste, and is malarial. It cleanses the blood, supports liver health, enhances the immune response, is a natural contraceptive, promotes faster wound healing, is effective against ulcers and gastritis, regulates blood sugar levels, and has anti-cancer properties.

- **Side effects**: skin rashes, itching, nausea, and diarrhea

- **Native habitat**: It originated from Asia but can be found in states like Florida, Mississippi, Texas, Louisiana, Hawaii,

Georgia, Alabama, Arizona, South Carolina, California, Puerto Rico, and the Virgin Islands.

- **Part(s) used**: leaves, bark, seeds, and oil

- **Preparation**: capsules, powders, oils, creams, and tinctures

- **Recommended dosage**: 500–1000 mg daily

- **Application methods**: You can take capsules with water or apply the oil topically.

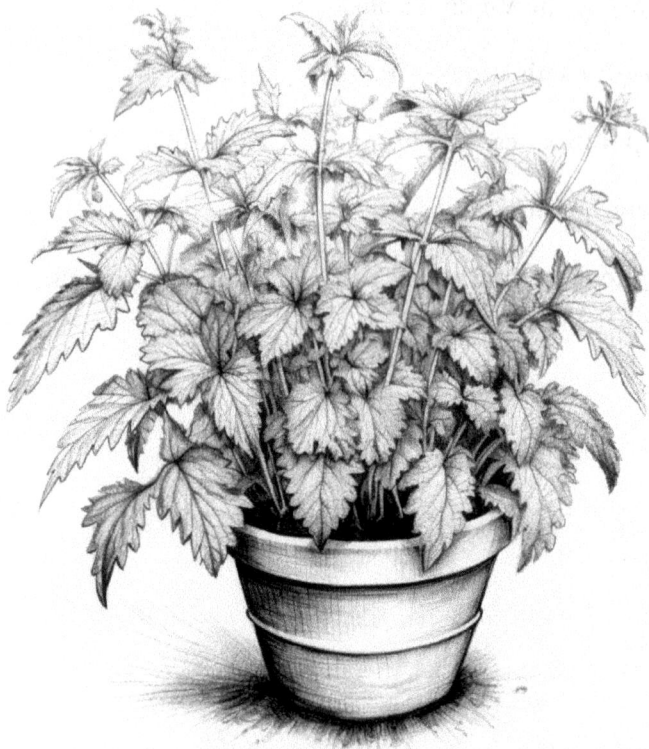

Nettle

- **Healing applications**: Nettle alleviates arthritis and joint pain, reduces symptoms of hay fever, supports kidney function and reduces fluid retention, promotes hair growth and reduces dandruff, is rich in iron, beneficial for those with anemia, eases muscle and menstrual pain, supports the management of benign prostatic hyperplasia (BPH), helps with allergic skin conditions, may aid in managing diabetes, enhances the immune system, assists in regulating blood pressure, is used for wound healing and bleeding control, alleviates digestive issues like indigestion, fights infections and supports overall health, and relieves symptoms of eczema.

- **Side effects**: skin rash, itching, upset stomach, or diarrhea.

- **Native habitat**: This herb is native to Europe, Asia, and North America. You can find it in Texas, New York, Florida, Oregon, California, Washington, Colorado, Illinois, Ohio, Pennsylvania, Michigan, Virginia, and more.

- **Part(s) used**: leaves and roots

- **Preparation**: teas, capsules, tinctures, and creams.

- **Recommended dosage**: 2–3 cups daily or the equivalent in grams for tinctures, oils, powders, and other extracts.

- **Application methods**: Make capsules and take them with water, or apply the oil topically. You can also brew tea with the leaves and roots of this plant or add its tincture to beverages and other foods.

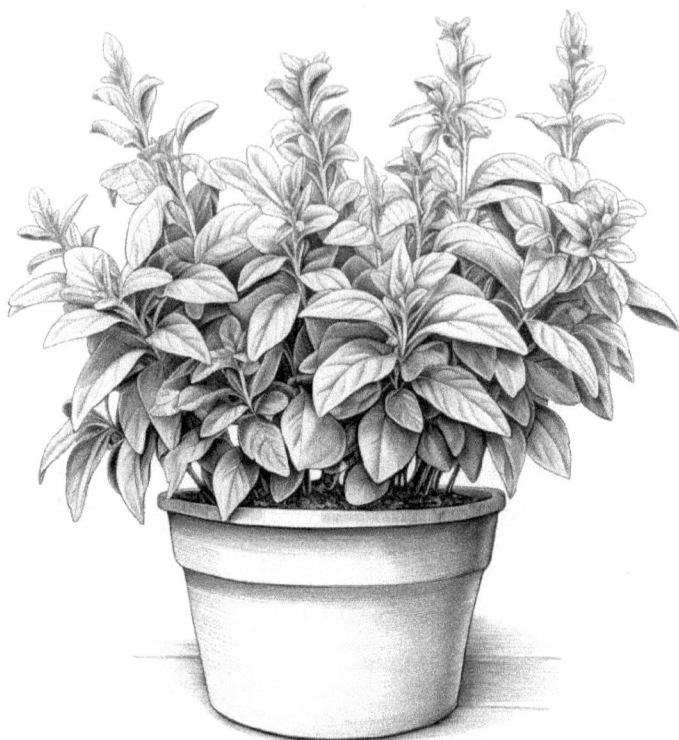

Nutmeg

- **Healing applications**: It eases indigestion and promotes
  digestion, alleviates muscle pain and joint pain, supports better
  sleep by inducing relaxation, reduces inflammation in various
  conditions, enhances memory and cognitive function, relieves
  respiratory issues like cough and asthma, assists in purifying the
  liver and kidneys, fights against bacterial infections, is used in
  toothpaste for its antimicrobial properties, acts as a natural
  relaxant, improves blood circulation in the body, alleviates
  menstrual cramps and discomfort, supports cardiovascular
  function, is a traditional remedy for nausea during pregnancy,
  and is used to enhance libido.

- **Side effects**: hallucinations, dizziness, skin rash, or swelling.

- **Native habitat**: It is native to Indonesia and grows in the following U.S. states: Puerto Rico, Florida, Texas, Hawaii, Louisiana, Georgia, Mississippi, Arizona, California, Alabama, South Carolina, and others.

- **Part(s) used**: seeds

- **Preparation**: essential oil, capsule, and tincture

- **Recommended dosage**: 1/4 to 1/2 teaspoon daily for powder

- **Application methods**: People usually consume the seeds by adding them to foods and beverages.

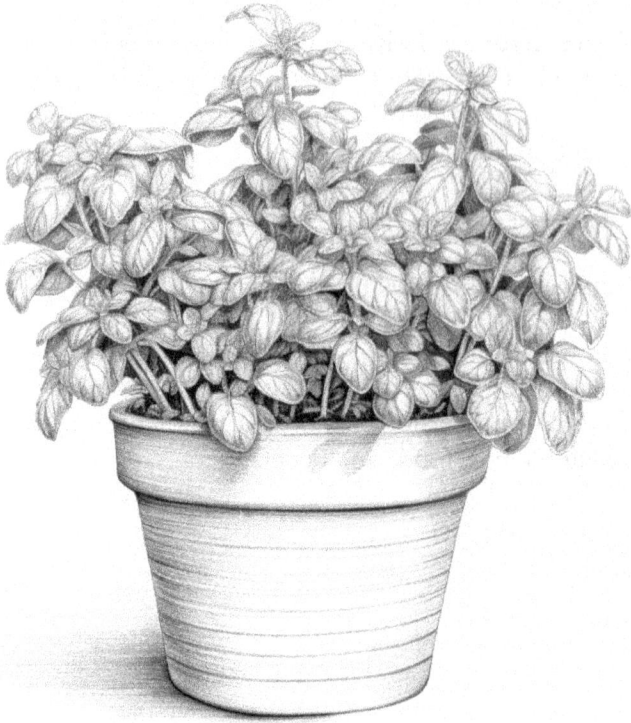

Oregano

- **Healing applications**: It fights against bacterial infections, reduces inflammation in various conditions, protects cells from oxidative stress, relieves symptoms of cough and asthma, eases indigestion and bloating, treats fungal infections like athlete's foot, alleviates muscle and joint pain, supports the immune system against viruses, eases menstrual cramps, is used topically for conditions like acne, supports cardiovascular function, helps with allergy symptoms, assists in reducing fluid retention, and is traditionally used to combat parasites, and fights cancer.

- **Side effects**: skin rash, itching, upset stomach, and diarrhea

- **Native habitat**: Native to the Mediterranean region, it also grows in California, Texas, Florida, Arizona, New Mexico, Nevada, Oregon, Washington, Colorado, Utah, Idaho, and Montana.

- **Part(s) used**: leaves and flowers

- **Preparation**: essential oil, capsules, tinctures, and powder

- **Recommended dosage**: 1–3 oil drops, depending on the concentration

- **Application methods**: Take the powder in tea or other beverages. You can also add it to your soup.

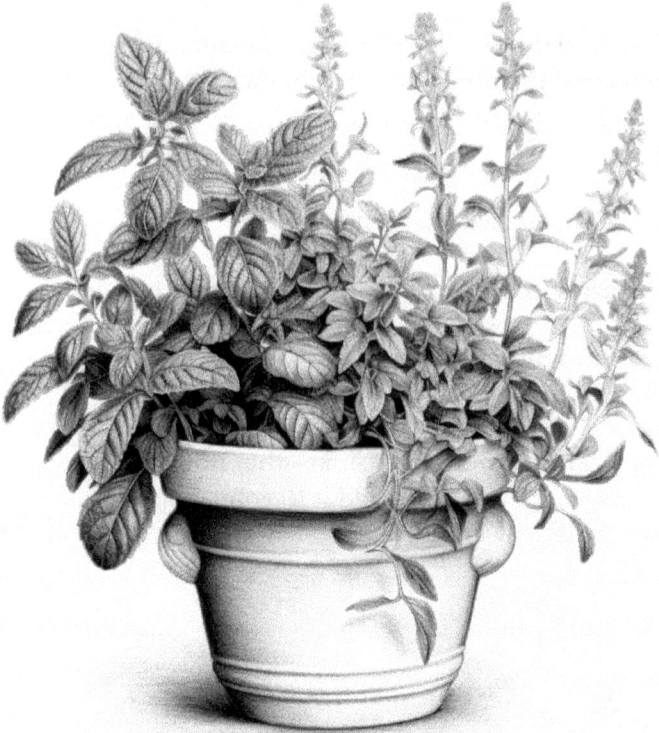

Paprika

- **Healing applications**: It reduces inflammation in joints and muscles, aids digestion and alleviates indigestion, supports overall health by combating oxidative stress, contains compounds beneficial for cardiovascular function, and may help in reducing pain, especially related to inflammation; some studies suggest a role in managing diabetes, used traditionally for respiratory conditions, exhibits antibacterial properties, may assist in weight loss efforts, contains compounds with potential anti-cancer effects, rich in carotenoids, beneficial for eye health, supports the immune system, used topically for skin conditions, some compounds may support brain health, and enhances the absorption of dietary iron.

- **Side effects**: skin rash, itching, upset stomach, or diarrhea when used excessively

- **Native habitat**: Native to Central America, this herb can be found in many states, including California, Pennsylvania, Texas, Florida, Arizona, Ohio, Georgia, South Carolina, Virginia, New Mexico, North Carolina, and Alabama.

- **Part(s) used**: fruit

- **Preparation**: Dry and grind the fruit for use as powder, tincture, and supplements.

- **Recommended dosage**: Use enough to spice up your dish.

- **Application methods**: Use the fruit as a spice in cooking or consume it whole.

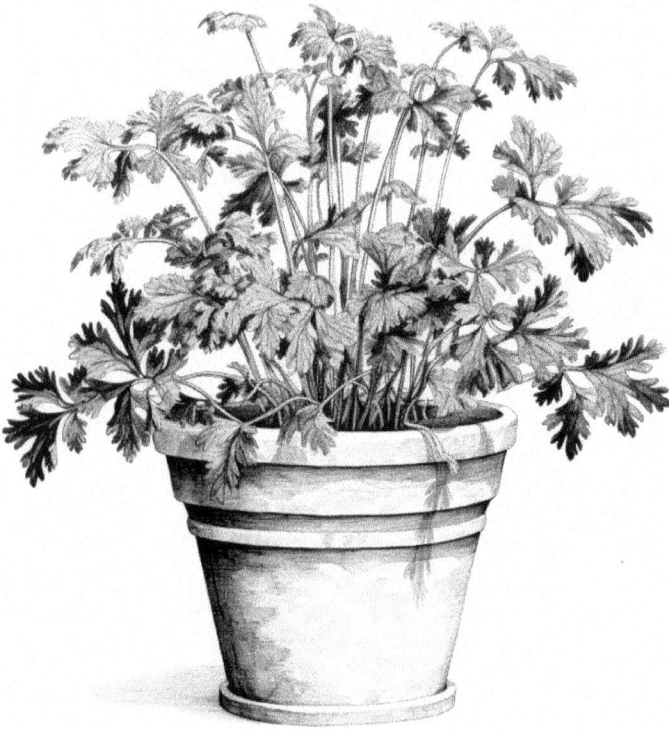

Parsley

- **Healing applications**: It reduces inflammation in conditions like arthritis, alleviates indigestion and bloating, supports kidney function and reduces fluid retention, is rich in antioxidants, promotes overall health, enhances the immune system, contains compounds with potential anti-cancer properties, is rich in vitamin K, vital for bone health, supports cardiovascular function, acts as a natural breath freshener, may help regulate menstrual cycles, contains nutrients beneficial for eye health, exhibits antibacterial properties, contains compounds that may help reduce anxiety, some studies suggest a role in managing diabetes, and may assist in lowering blood pressure.

- **Side effects**: skin rash or itching. It's not good for people with kidney disease, as it may worsen it.

- **Native habitat**: You can find this plant in California, Texas, Florida, New York, Pennsylvania, Illinois, Ohio, Michigan, Georgia, North Carolina, Virginia, Arizona, and other states.

- **Part(s) used**: leaves, stems, and roots

- **Preparation**: tinctures, tea, oil, and dried flakes

- **Recommended dosage**: Use as much as necessary in your recipes or meals.

- **Application methods**: It is usually eaten in salads or used for preparing food.

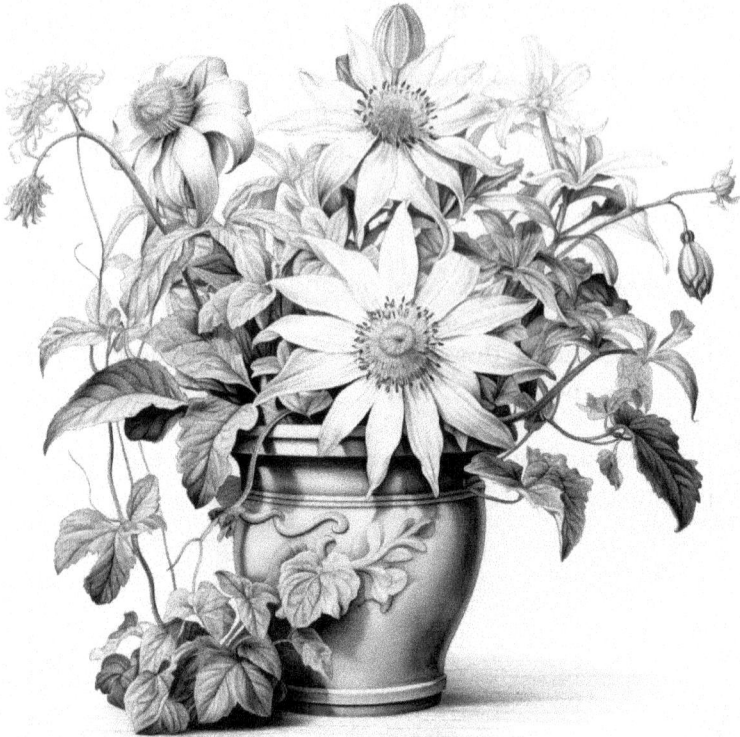

Passionflower

- **Healing applications**: It calms the nervous system and reduces anxiety, helps with insomnia and promotes restful sleep, acts as a natural stress reliever, alleviates discomfort and muscle tension, reduces inflammation in certain conditions, may help lower blood pressure, supports overall health by combating oxidative stress, eases menstrual cramps and discomfort, supports brain health and cognitive function, is used for gastrointestinal issues like indigestion, is traditionally used for respiratory conditions, relieves muscle spasms and cramps, helps alleviate premenstrual syndrome symptoms, is used in managing withdrawal symptoms, and may have potential in managing seizures.

- **Side effects**: drowsiness, nausea, stomach upset

- **Native habitat**: Look for this plant in all U.S. states, including Florida, Texas, Georgia, North Carolina, South Carolina, Virginia, Alabama, Mississippi, Louisiana, Arkansas, Oklahoma, and Tennessee.

- **Part(s) used**: leaves, stems, and flowers.

- **Preparation**: teas, tinctures, powder, chemical extracts

- **Recommended dosage**: 1–2 teaspoons of powder or its equivalent in tinctures

- **Application methods**: You can take the ground form in tea and other beverages or drink the tincture directly.

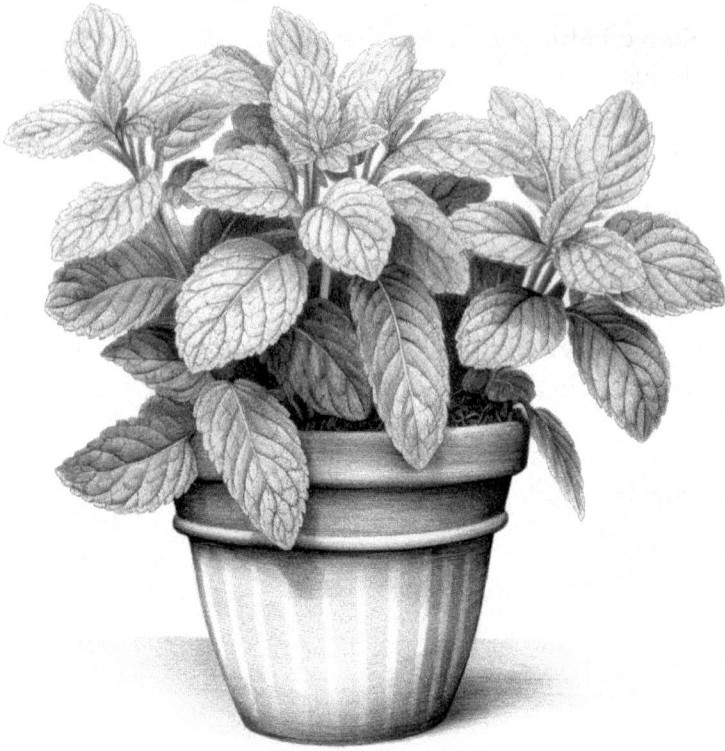

Peppermint

- **Healing applications**: It relieves indigestion and bloating, eases
  tension headaches, soothes symptoms of colds and congestion,
  alleviates nausea and motion sickness, relieves muscle spasms
  and cramps, reduces discomfort, including menstrual pain, acts
  as a natural stress reliever, has a cooling effect that may help
  reduce fever, exhibits antibacterial properties, alleviates
  inflammation in various conditions, aids in concentration and
  mental clarity, may help with allergy symptoms, is used topically
  for conditions like itching, supports the immune system, and is
  used in some weight loss efforts.

- **Side effects**: may cause heartburn, skin rash, or itching

- **Native habitat**: Originated from Europe and the Middle East but grows in several American states such as Washington, Oregon, Idaho, Indiana, Michigan, Wisconsin, New York, Pennsylvania, Ohio, Oregon, and Montana.

- **Part(s) used**: leaves and stems

- **Preparation**: teas, essential oil, capsules, and tinctures

- **Recommended dosage**: 1–2 teaspoons dried leaves

- **Application methods**: You can take it in the form of tinctures or tea but also apply it topically as a cream.

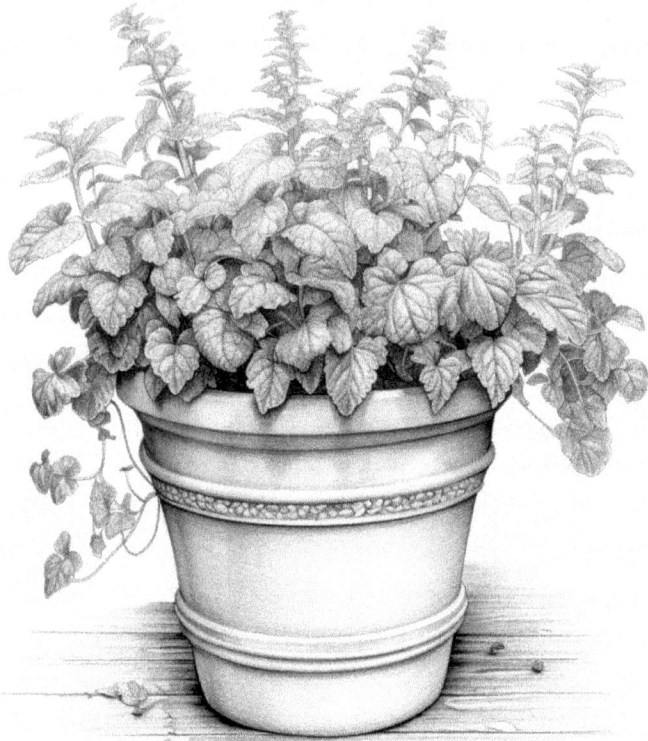

Perilla

- **Healing applications**: It reduces inflammation in conditions like arthritis, may alleviate symptoms of hay fever, is used in traditional medicine for asthma, supports overall health by combating oxidative stress, eases indigestion and bloating, may help with respiratory conditions, exhibits antibacterial properties, some compounds may support brain health, may aid in weight loss efforts, some studies suggest potential cancer-fighting effects, is used traditionally for managing diabetes, contains compounds that may help reduce anxiety, supports heart health, fights against various microbial infections, and is used topically for conditions like dermatitis.

- **Side effects**: Skin rash, itching, upset stomach, and diarrhea may occur when you take too much of this herb.

- **Native habitat**: This herb originated in East Asia and now grows in California, Texas, New York, Georgia, Florida, North Carolina, Virginia, Maryland, Oregon, Washington, Hawaii, Massachusetts, and other states.

- **Part(s) used**: leaves and seeds

- **Preparation:** teas, tinctures, capsules, and an oil

- **Recommended dosage**: 1–2 teaspoons dry leaves or its equivalent in tinctures and teas

- **Application methods**: Use the leaves to brew tea or use the oil in food.

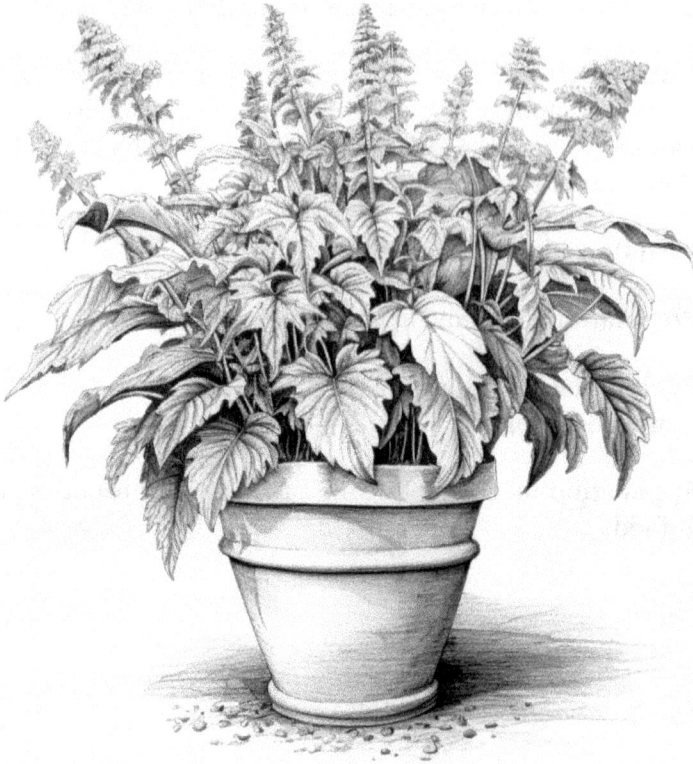

Plantain

- **Healing applications**: Used topically for cuts and wounds, reduces inflammation in skin conditions, eases respiratory symptoms, alleviates digestive issues like indigestion, exhibits antibacterial properties, is used for conditions like eczema and dermatitis, supports kidney function and reduces fluid retention, fights against microbial infections, soothes minor burns and sunburn, helps with allergy symptoms, is used for issues like gastritis, provides relief from insect bites, soothes and reduces throat irritation, supports the immune system, and is traditionally used for hemorrhoids.

- **Side effects**: Skin rash, itching, upset stomach, and diarrhea are some allergies that may occur, especially when you take high doses.

- **Native habitat**: Native to Europe, it also grows in states like California, Texas, Florida, New York, Ohio, North Carolina, Virginia, Georgia, Michigan, Pennsylvania, Illinois, and Massachusetts.

- **Part(s) used**: leaves, roots, and seeds

- **Preparation**: tinctures, powders, oils, teas

- **Recommended dosage**: 1–2 teaspoons for teas

- **Application methods**: People usually consume this herb in the form of tea or directly as a tincture. You can also add the tincture to your beverages and other snacks.

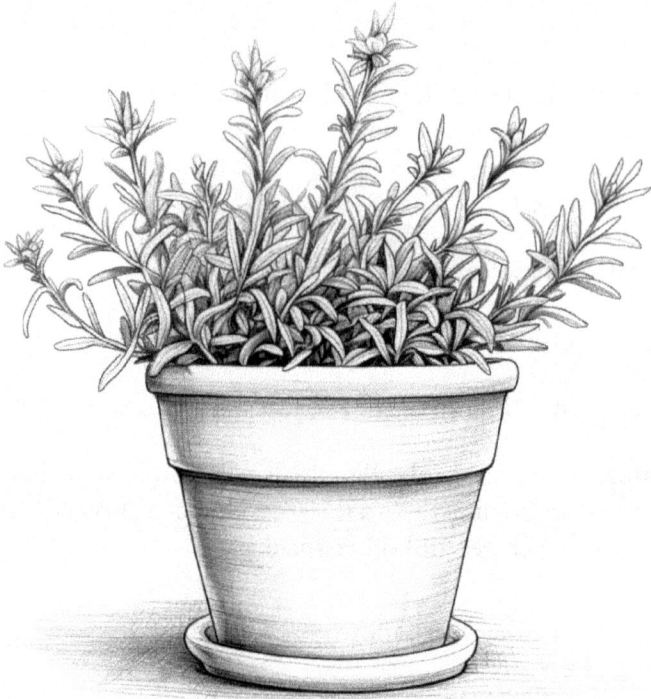

Rosemary

- **Healing applications**: It supports memory and concentration, reduces inflammation in various conditions, eases indigestion and bloating, is used for respiratory issues like congestion, supports overall health, alleviates muscle pain and headaches, exhibits antibacterial properties, promotes hair growth and reduces dandruff, acts as a natural stress reliever, enhances blood circulation, some studies suggest potential cancer-fighting effects, supports the immune system, is used topically for conditions like eczema, eases menstrual cramps, and is used for arthritis and joint pain.

- **Side effects**: Skin rash, itching, upset stomach, or diarrhea are some allergies that may occur especially when you take high doses.

- **Native habitat**: Native to the Mediterranean region, it also grows in states like California, Texas, Florida, Arizona, New Mexico, Georgia, North Carolina, Virginia, Oregon, Washington, Alabama, and South Carolina.

- **Part(s) used**: leaves and flowers

- **Preparation**: oils, teas, tinctures, and powders

- **Recommended dosage**: 1–2 teaspoons for tea

- **Application methods**: People usually consume this herb in the form of tea or directly as a tincture. You can also add the tincture to your beverages and other snacks. Apply externally for aromatherapy.

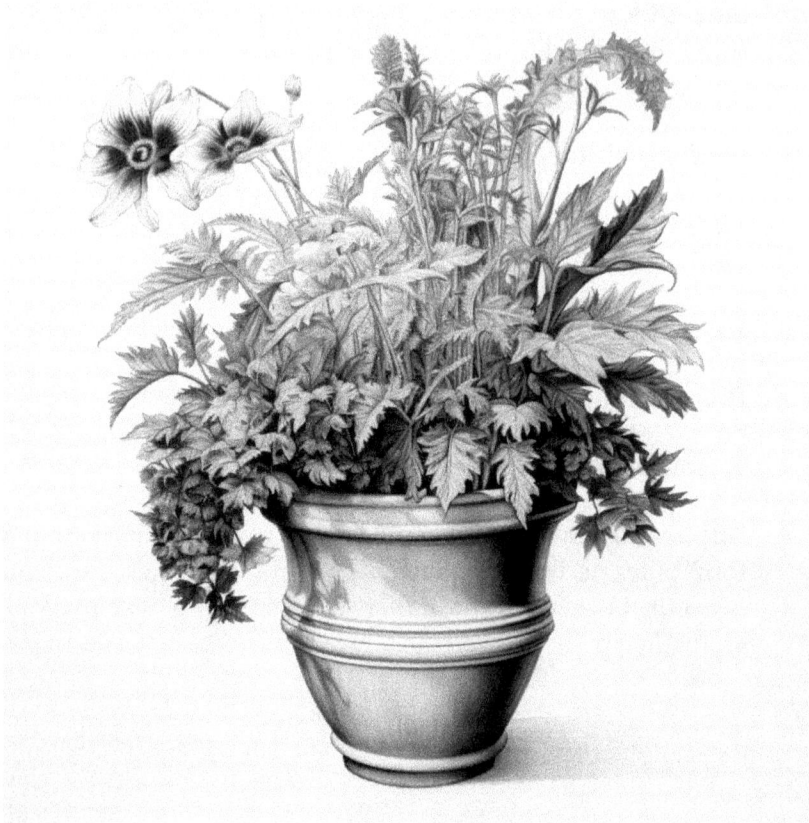

Saffron

- **Healing applications**: It alleviates symptoms of depression, is used to reduce inflammation in various conditions, is believed to improve cognitive function and memory, is traditionally used for enhancing libido and treating sexual disorders, some studies suggest saffron may have anti-cancer properties, rich in antioxidants that combat oxidative stress, used to alleviate symptoms of premenstrual syndrome, may aid in respiratory conditions like asthma, saffron may contribute to heart health, traditionally used for digestive issues, believed to have sleep-inducing properties, some studies suggest saffron may help regulate blood sugar, applied topically for skin health and anti-aging effects, used for its analgesic properties, and potential benefits for neurodegenerative conditions

- **Side effects**: An upset stomach and diarrhea are some allergies that may occur especially when you take high doses.

- **Native habitat**: Native to Southwest Asia, it also grows in states like California, Pennsylvania, Vermont, New York, Connecticut, Michigan, Oregon, Washington, Colorado, New Mexico, Arizona, and Texas.

- **Part(s) used**: the red stigmas from the flowers

- **Preparation**: tinctures, powders, oils, teas

- **Recommended dosage**: 20 mg to 100 mg per day

- **Application methods**: People usually consume this herb in the form of tea or directly as a tincture. You can also add the tincture to your beverages and other snacks.

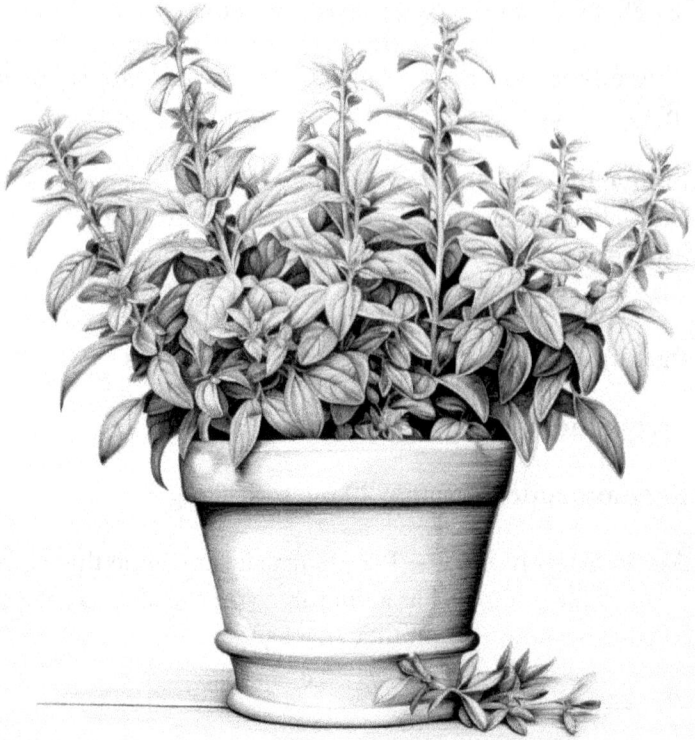

Sage

- **Healing applications**: It enhances memory and cognitive function, is used to reduce inflammation in conditions like arthritis, traditionally used to alleviate digestive issues; sage has antimicrobial properties, is often used for throat infections, and is known to alleviate hot flashes and hormonal imbalances, some studies suggest sage may help regulate blood sugar, used for its calming effects on the nervous system, sage may help with mouth and throat infections, applied topically for its antimicrobial properties, sage has been used for coughs and respiratory infections, some studies suggest it may help lower blood pressure, rich in antioxidants that combat oxidative stress, may provide relief from allergic reactions, some research suggests sage may have anti-cancer properties, and used traditionally for various types of pain.

- **Side effects**: digestive discomfort and diarrhea are some allergies that may occur especially when you take high doses.

- **Native habitat**: Native to the Mediterranean region, it also grows in states like California, Oregon, Washington, Idaho, Nevada, Utah, Arizona, New Mexico, Colorado, Wyoming, Montana, Texas, and more.

- **Part(s) used**: leaves

- **Preparation**: tinctures, powders, oils, teas

- **Recommended dosage**: 300 mg to 600 mg daily

- **Application methods**: People usually consume this herb in the form of tea, in food, or directly as a tincture. You can also add the tincture to your beverages and other snacks.

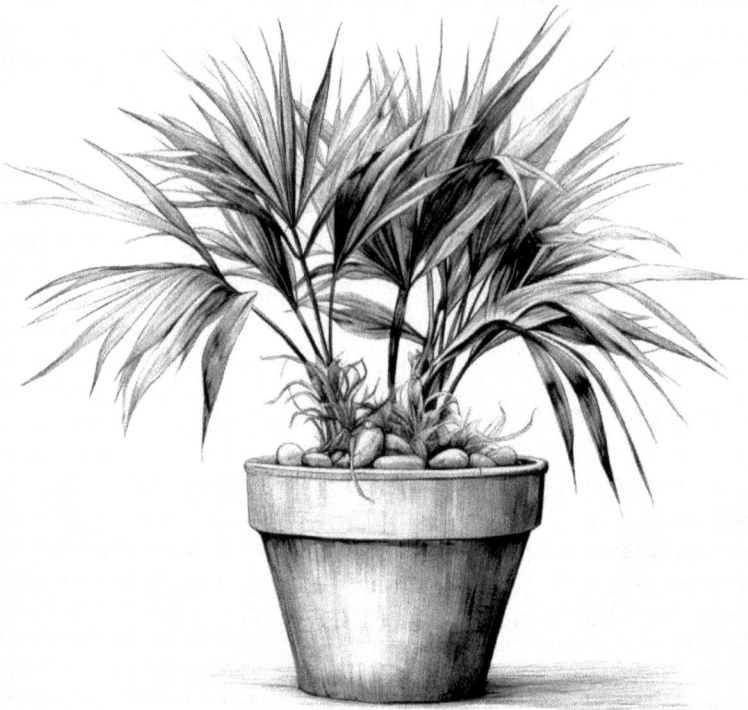

Saw Palmetto

- **Healing applications**: It is commonly used to alleviate symptoms of benign prostatic hyperplasia (BPH), saw palmetto may support urinary function in men, used to address hormonal imbalances, especially in women; some use it to promote hair growth and prevent hair loss, saw palmetto has anti-inflammatory properties, believed to enhance libido and sexual function, traditional use for respiratory issues, saw palmetto may support reproductive health in men, used for its potential benefits in respiratory infections, potential use in conditions related to androgen excess, saw palmetto may have positive effects on bladder function, some use it for its potential in reducing migraines, applied topically, it may benefit skin conditions like acne, some studies suggest saw palmetto may aid in diabetes management, and saw palmetto may have calming effects on the nervous system

- **Side effects**: Headache and stomach upsets are some allergies that may occur, especially when you take high doses.

- **Native habitat**: Native to the southeastern United States, it grows in states like Florida, Georgia, Alabama, Mississippi, Louisiana, South Carolina, North Carolina, Texas, Arkansas, Virginia, Tennessee, Kentucky, and others.

- **Part(s) used**: ripe berries

- **Preparation**: tinctures, powders, and teas

- **Recommended dosage**: 160 mg to 320 mg daily

- **Application methods**: People usually consume these berries with food, alone, or as supplements.

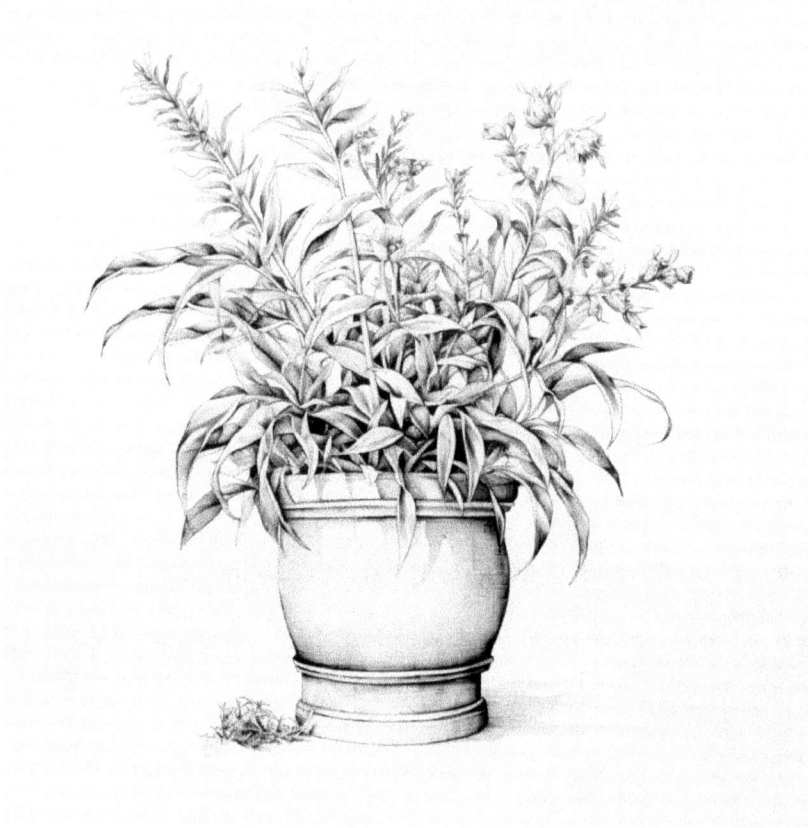

Sea Buckthorn

- **Healing applications**: This herb is rich in vitamin C, supports immune function, potential benefits for heart health and cholesterol levels, used for wounds, burns, and skin conditions, may help reduce inflammation in various conditions, traditionally used for gastrointestinal issues, contains nutrients beneficial for vision, some studies suggest sea buckthorn may aid liver function, potential use in weight loss regimens, used for respiratory conditions like asthma, some research indicates anti-cancer properties, potential benefits for arthritis and joint pain, used for hormonal balance and menopausal symptoms, rich in antioxidants combating oxidative stress, some studies suggest sea buckthorn may help manage diabetes, and used for improving hair and nail condition.

- **Side effects**: Stomach upset and inflated blood pressure are some allergies that may occur, especially when you take high doses.

- **Native habitat**: Native to Europe and Asia, it also grows in states like Alaska, Washington, Oregon, California, Idaho, Montana, Wyoming, Colorado, Utah, Nevada, New Mexico, and Arizona.

- **Part(s) used**: seeds and berries

- **Preparation**: tinctures, powders, oils, teas

- **Recommended dosage**: 300 mg to 2000 mg daily

- **Application methods**: People usually consume these berries and oils from the seeds in foods or directly.

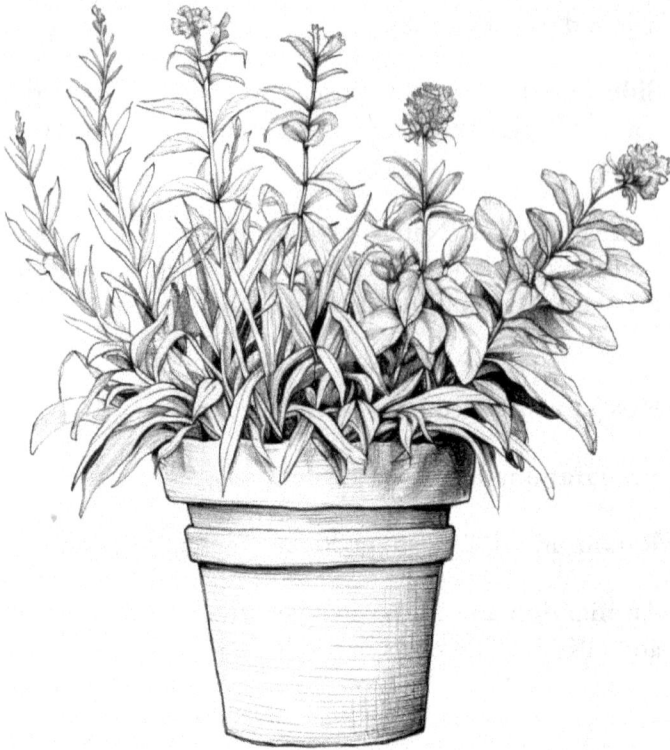

Sida

- **Healing applications**: It is used to alleviate inflammation in conditions like arthritis, is a traditional remedy for respiratory issues, is used for gastrointestinal problems, may help manage diarrhea, is rich in antioxidants that combat oxidative stress, is traditionally used for reducing fever, is used for various types of pain relief, is a traditional remedy for UTIs, may have antimicrobial properties, is applied topically for wounds and skin infections, some studies suggest sida may help regulate blood sugar, research indicates potential anti-cancer properties, traditional use for calming effects on the nervous system, treating asthma and bronchitis, and modulating the immune system.

- **Side effects**: stomach upset, and low blood pressure are some allergies that may occur, especially when you take high doses.

- **Native habitat**: It is found worldwide and grows in states like Florida, Texas, California, Louisiana, Mississippi, Alabama, Georgia, South Carolina, North Carolina, Virginia, Maryland, Delaware and more.

- **Part(s) used**: leaves and seeds

- **Preparation:** tinctures, powders, oils, teas, infusions

- **Recommended dosage**: This herb is banned in the U.S., but we see traces of it in supplements.

- **Application methods**: People usually consume this herb in the form of tea or directly as a tincture or infusion. You can also use it topically for skincare.

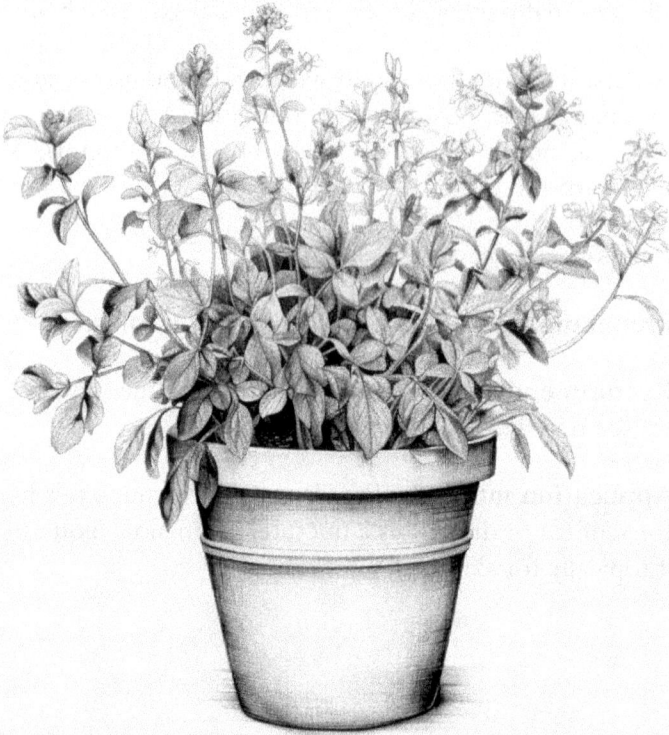

Soy

- **Healing applications**: Soy may lower cholesterol levels, reducing the risk of cardiovascular disease, isoflavones in soy can help manage menopausal symptoms, soy is rich in nutrients supporting bone density, some studies suggest soy may reduce the risk of certain cancers, soy protein can aid in weight loss and muscle building, soy may help manage diabetes and improve insulin sensitivity, soy fiber supports gastrointestinal health, isoflavones exhibit anti-inflammatory properties, phytoestrogens in soy may help balance hormones, soy-based products can benefit skin conditions, soy consumption may affect thyroid hormone levels positively, antioxidants in soy may protect against age-related macular degeneration, soy may reduce symptoms in asthma patients, soy proteins may aid in liver function, and soy peptides may enhance immune response.

- **Side effects**: Itching and swelling are some allergies that may occur, especially when you take high doses.

- **Native habitat**: Native to East Asia, it also grows in states like Iowa, Illinois, Minnesota, Nebraska, Indiana, Ohio, South Dakota, Missouri, Arkansas, North Dakota, Kansas, and Mississippi.

- **Part(s) used**: seeds

- **Preparation**: powders, oil, and soy-based food products

- **Recommended dosage**: 25 gram daily

- **Application methods**: People usually consume soybeans incorporated into their diets.

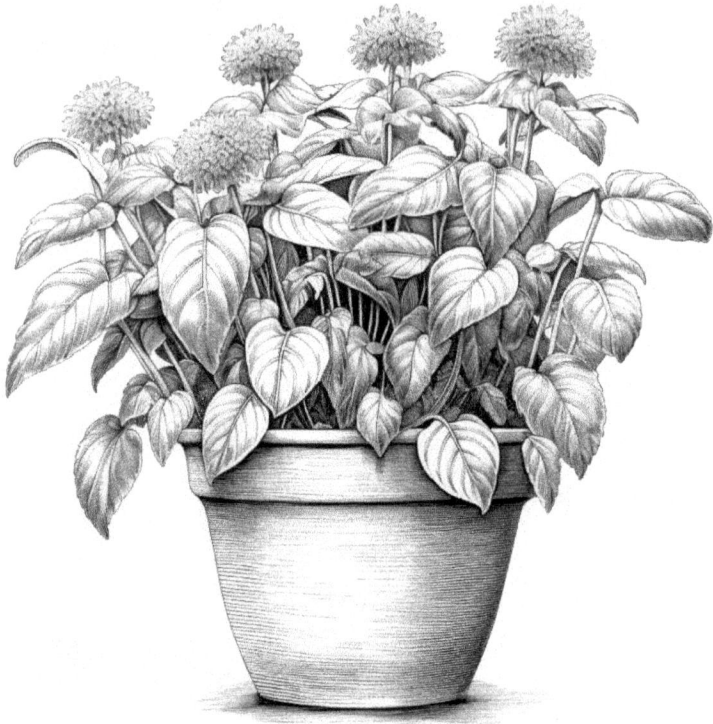

Spilanthes

- **Healing applications**: It is used for toothaches and gum issues, fights infections like candida, enhances overall immunity, alleviates inflammation, treats colds and respiratory infections, eases digestive discomfort, combats intestinal parasites, is used to enhance libido, acts as a natural analgesic, promotes urine flow, is effective against fungal infections, treats eczema and dermatitis, targets certain viruses, lowers body temperature, and is investigated for potential anti-cancer effects.

- **Side effects**: some potential adverse reactions to this herb are

- **Native habitat**: It originated in South America and grows in many states, including Florida, Texas, California, Louisiana,

Mississippi, Alabama, Georgia, South Carolina, North Carolina, Virginia, Maryland, and Delaware.

- **Part(s) used**: leaves and flowers

- **Preparation**: Tinctures, infusions, oils, and powders

- **Recommended dosage**: 1 to 3 ml of tincture or 1 to 2 cups of tea daily

- **Application methods**: There are several ways to take this herb. You can drink the tincture or add it to a beverage. You can also steep the dried version in hot water or brew tea with it.

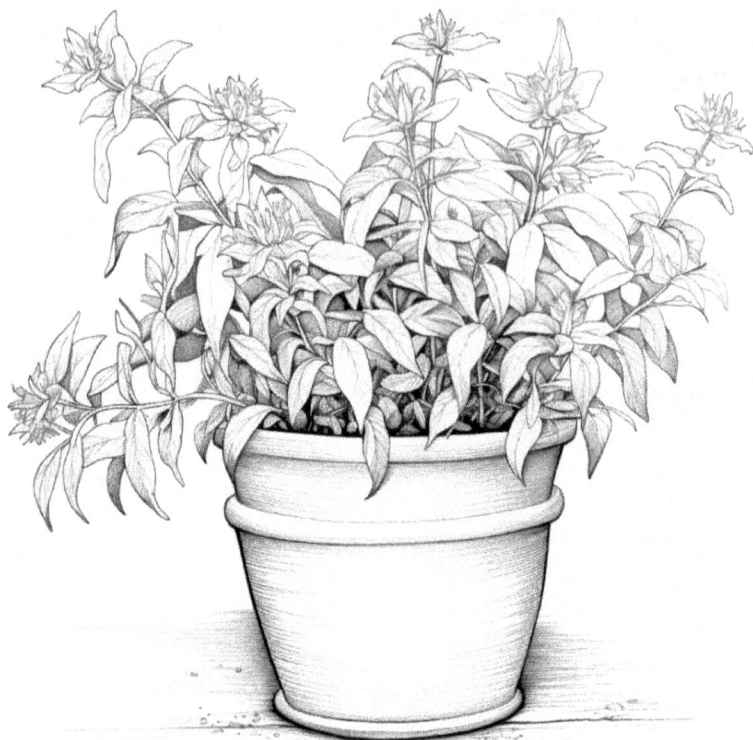

St John's Wort

- **Healing applications**: The herb eases mild to moderate depression, alleviates symptoms of anxiety, helps improve sleep quality, accelerates the healing process, reduces inflammation, alleviates neuropathic pain, may reduce symptoms, addresses mood swings and irritability, manages symptoms like mood changes, exhibits antiviral properties, is used for certain bacterial infections, treats wounds, burns, and skin irritations, may help manage symptoms, mitigates winter blues, and supports digestive health.

- **Side effects**: Sensitivity to sunlight and metabolic effects. Some potential adverse reactions to this herb are

- **Native habitat**: It originated in Europe, Asia, and North Africa and grows in many states, including California, Oregon, Washington, Idaho, Montana, Wyoming, Colorado, Utah, Arizona, New Mexico, Texas, and Arkansas.

- **Part(s) used**: the flowering tops

- **Preparation**: capsules, tinctures, teas, and refined extracts

- **Recommended dosage**: 300 to 900 mg daily

- **Application methods**: There are several ways to take this herb. You can drink the tincture or add it to a beverage. You can also steep the dried version in hot water or brew tea with it.

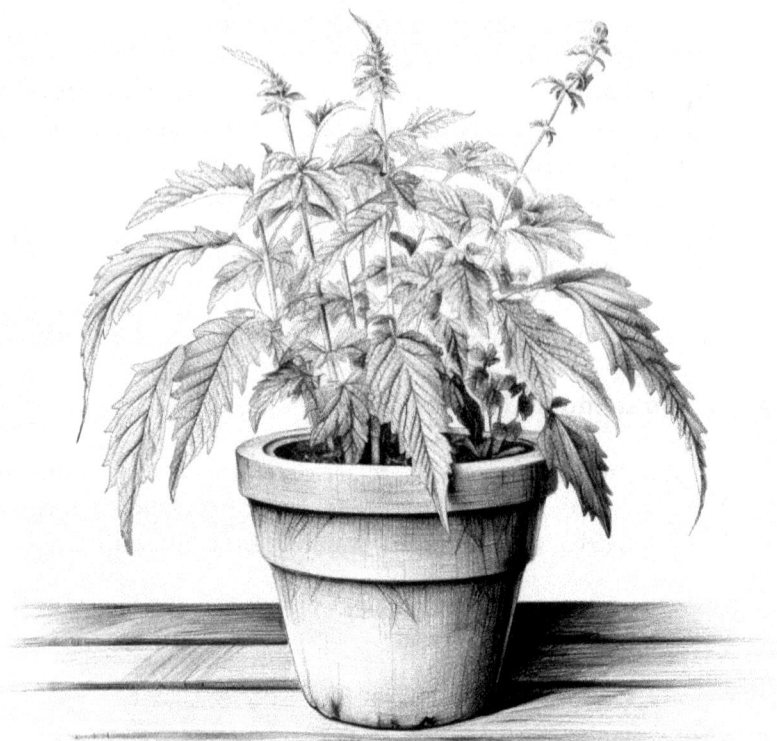

Stinging Nettle

- **Healing applications**: It alleviates hay fever symptoms, reduces inflammation in joints, relieves symptoms of rheumatoid arthritis, boosts iron levels in the blood, aids in flushing out toxins, supports a healthy prostate, may help regulate glucose levels, acts as a natural hypotensive, soothes skin conditions, assists in urinary issues, eases joint pain in osteoarthritis, promotes hair growth and scalp health, reduces symptoms of PMS, addresses allergic rhinitis symptoms, and nettle leaves are rich in protein.

- **Side effects**: Rashes and upset stomach are some potential drawbacks of using this herb.

- **Native habitat**: It originated from Europe and Asia, and also grows in California, Oregon, Washington, Montana, Idaho, Wyoming, Colorado, Utah, Arizona, New Mexico, Texas, Arkansas, and other states.

- **Part(s) used**: leaves, stems, and roots

- **Preparation**: teas, capsules, tinctures, and purified extracts

- **Recommended dosage**: 300–600 mg of dried leaf or 2–4 ml of tincture daily

- **Application methods**: It is usually taken orally as tea or by taking the tinctures and infusions directly. You can also use it as an ingredient in your recipes.

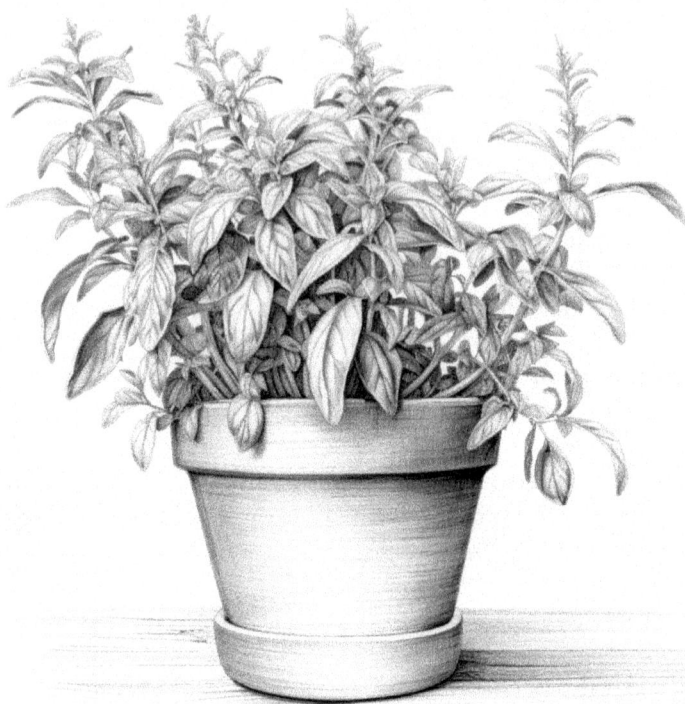

Tarragon

- **Healing applications**: The herb alleviates indigestion and flatulence, boosts appetite, relieves insomnia symptoms, fights certain bacterial infections, reduces inflammation, eases toothaches and joint pain, alleviates menstrual cramps, supports urine flow, used for gum and mouth issues, calms nervousness and anxiety, may help manage symptoms, assists in regulating glucose levels, soothes coughs, addresses hay fever symptoms, and supports the body's detox processes.

- **Side effects**: Some potential adverse reactions to this herb are stomach upset and diarrhea.

- **Native habitat**: It originated in Eurasia and grows in many U.S. states, including California, Oregon, Washington, Montana, Idaho, Wyoming, Colorado, Utah, Arizona, New Mexico, Texas, Louisiana, and others.

- **Part(s) used**: leaves and stems

- **Preparation**: teas, tinctures, and refined extracts

- **Recommended dosage**: It is safe to take in food amounts

- **Application methods**: There are several ways to do it. You can drink the tincture or add it to a beverage. You can also steep the dried version in hot water or brew tea with it.

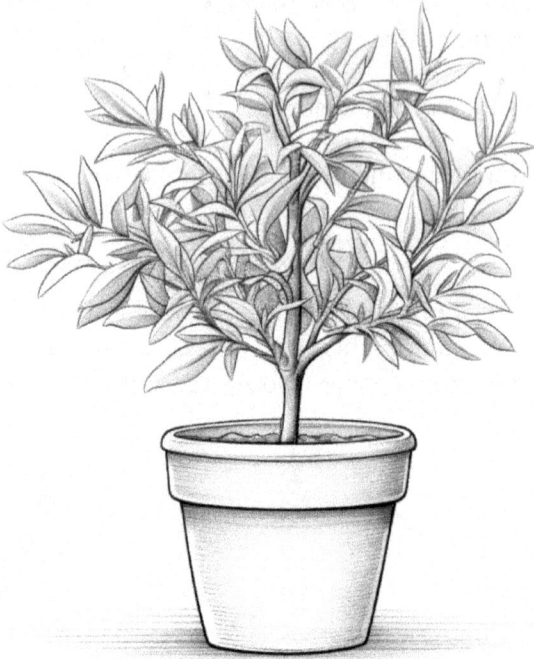

Tea Tree

- **Healing applications**: This herb treats skin infections and wounds, combats fungal infections like athlete's foot, helps manage viral infections, reduces acne and blemishes, addresses scalp conditions, soothes itching and inflammation, eases congestion and coughs, boosts the immune system, accelerates wound recovery, acts as a natural deodorant, aids in relieving sinusitis symptoms, supports oral health, reduces inflammation, alleviates muscle aches, and manages candidiasis.

- **Side effects**: Some potential adverse reactions to this herb are gynecomastia and irritation.

- **Native habitat**: It originated in Australia and grows in many states, including California, Texas, Florida, Arizona, Louisiana, Georgia, Alabama, Mississippi, South Carolina, North Carolina, Virginia, Hawaii, and others.

- **Part(s) used**: leaves and trees

- **Preparation:** essential oil, creams, ointments, shampoos, and diluted solutions (5–10% strength).

- **Recommended dosage**: 3–4 cups of tea daily

- **Application methods**: There are several ways to take this herb. You can drink the leaves tincture or add it to a beverage. Its oil is applied topically only.

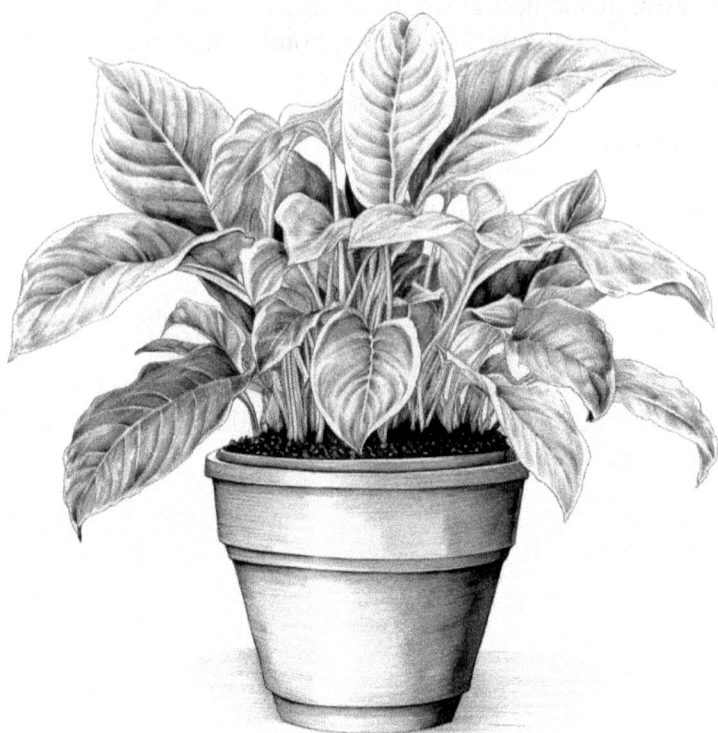

Turmeric

- **Healing applications**: Turmeric is effective against inflammation in arthritis, protects cells from oxidative stress, aids in digestion and reduces bloating, supports liver function, helps manage cholesterol levels, is investigated for potential anti-cancer properties, accelerates wound recovery, may support cognitive function, helps regulate blood sugar, has potential mood-enhancing effects, addresses psoriasis and eczema, supports weight loss efforts, alleviates pain in conditions like osteoarthritis, may reduce symptoms, and assists in managing respiratory issues.

- **Side effects**: Some potential adverse reactions to this herb are stomach upset and diarrhea.

- **Native habitat**: It originated in South Asia and grows in many states, including Florida, Texas, California, Hawaii, Louisiana, Georgia, Alabama, Mississippi, South Carolina, North Carolina, Virginia, Maryland, and others.

- **Part(s) used**: stems and rhizomes

- **Preparation**: capsules, powders, tinctures, and teas

- **Recommended dosage**: 500 to 2,000 mg daily

- **Application methods**: There are several ways to take this herb. You can drink the tincture, add it to tea, or use it as an ingredient in cooking. Add some pepper to maximize absorption.

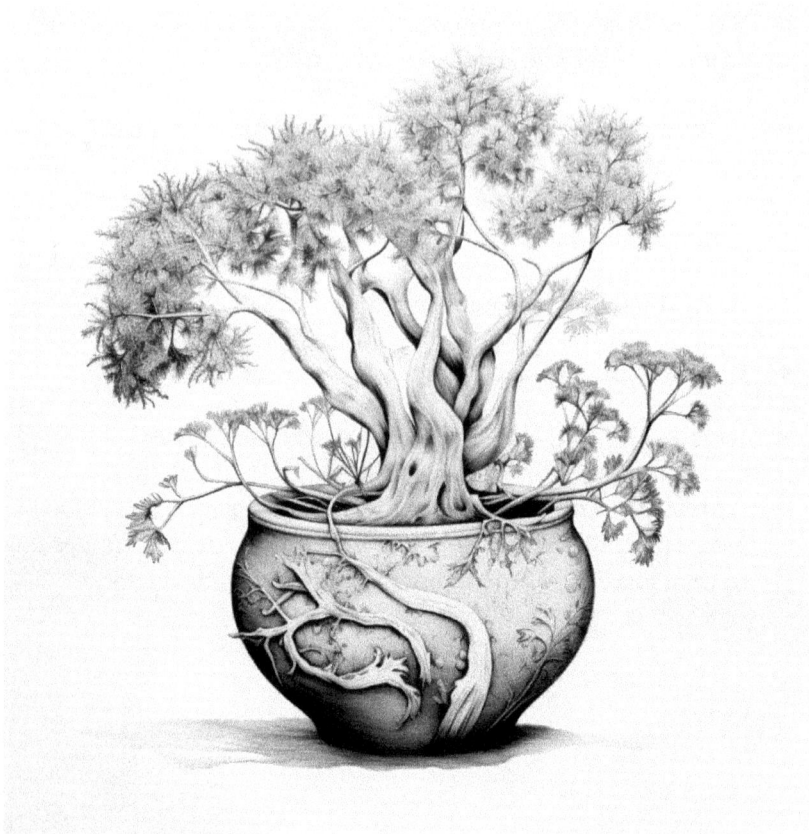

Usnea

- **Healing applications**: It fights bacterial infections, addresses viral infections like the flu, reduces inflammation, aids in bronchial conditions, boosts the immune system, accelerates wound recovery, combats UTIs, is used for gum and mouth issues, lowers body temperature, eases sinusitis symptoms, soothes persistent coughs, addresses sore throats, treats fungal infections, is investigated for potential benefits, and addresses certain parasites.

- **Side effects**: Some potential adverse reactions to this herb are skin irritation and an upset stomach.

- **Native habitat**: It originated in North America and grows in many states, including Alaska, Washington, Oregon, California, Idaho, Montana, Wyoming, Colorado, New Mexico, Arizona, Utah, Nevada, and many others.

- **Part(s) used**: the thallus

- **Preparation**: Brew this herb into tea or use its tincture with beverages and other edibles. Apply the ointment topically.

- **Recommended dosage**: 500 mg to 2 grams daily

- **Application methods**: There are several ways to take this herb. You can drink the tincture or add it to a beverage. You can also steep the dried version in hot water or brew tea with it.

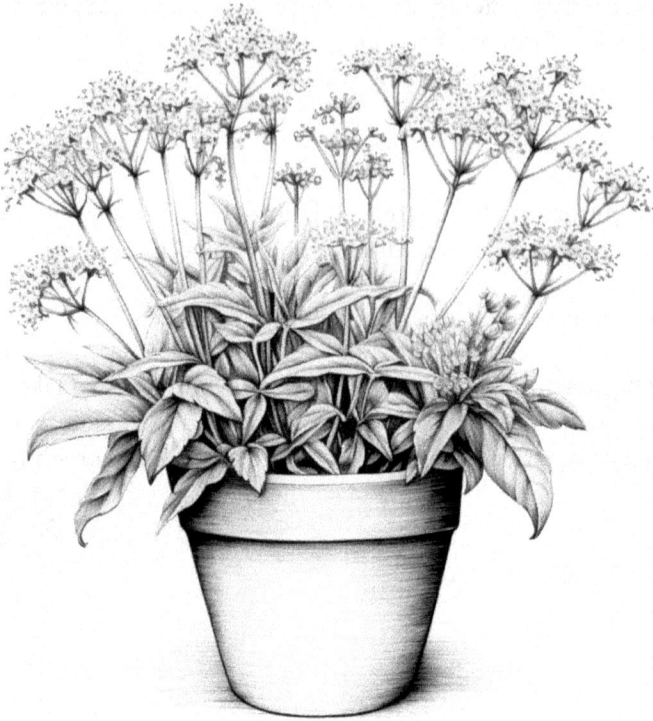

Valerian

- **Healing applications**: It aids in sleep disorders, calms nervousness and anxiety, alleviates stress-related symptoms, eases muscle tension, may reduce headache intensity, alleviates menstrual pain, eases digestive discomfort, may help lower blood pressure, supports focus in ADHD, assists in managing arthritis pain, is investigated for migraine relief, may ease symptoms, is used for respiratory issues, has potential benefits for neurological conditions, and is used for appetite enhancement.

- **Side effects**: Some potential adverse reactions to this herb are sleepiness and stomach discomfort.

- **Native habitat**: It originated in Europe and Asia and grows in many states, including California, Oregon, Washington, Montana, Idaho, Wyoming, Colorado, New Mexico, Arizona, Utah, Texas, and Missouri.

- **Part(s) used**: roots and rhizomes

- **Preparation**: Brew this herb into tea or use its tincture with beverages and other edibles. Apply the ointment topically.

- **Recommended dosage**: 300 to 600 mg just before bedtime

- **Application methods**: There are a few ways to take this herb. You can drink the tincture or add it to a beverage. You can also steep the dried version in hot water or brew tea with it.

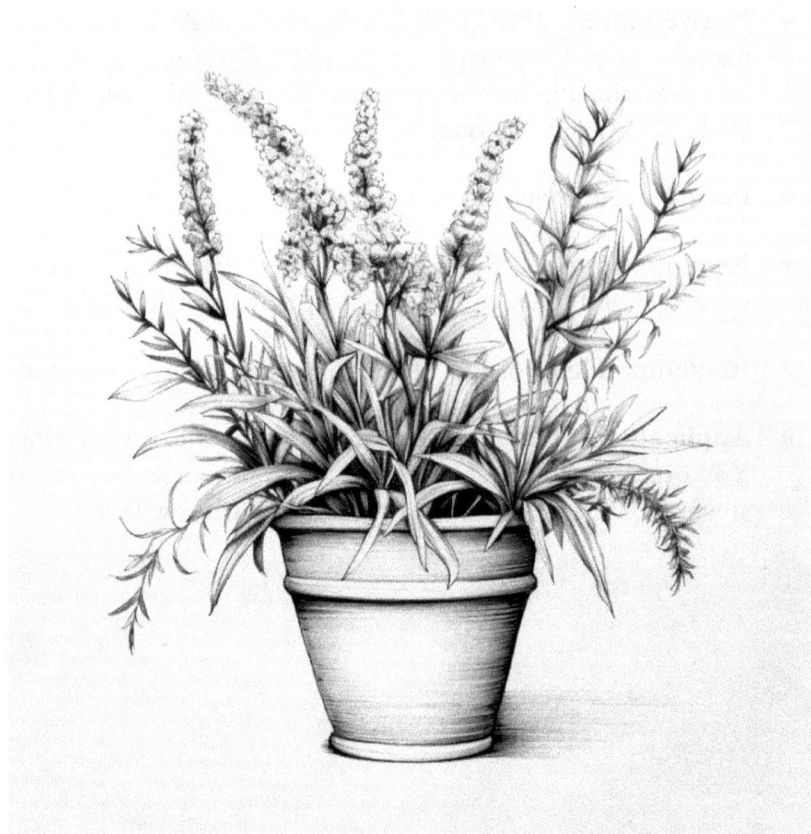

White Willow

- **Healing applications**: It acts as a natural analgesic, reduces inflammation, lowers body temperature, eases joint pain, alleviates tension headaches, reduces cramps, addresses lumbar discomfort, manages symptoms of osteoarthritis, relieves muscular aches, assists in gout symptom relief, may alleviate bursitis pain, is investigated for potential benefits, is used for toothaches, supports tendinitis management, and is topically applied for certain skin issues.

- **Side effects**: Some potential adverse reactions to this herb are stomach upset and diarrhea.

- **Native habitat**: It originated in Europe and Asia and also grows in many states, including Maine, New Hampshire, Vermont, Massachusetts, Connecticut, Rhode Island, New York, New Jersey, Pennsylvania, Maryland, West Virginia, and Ohio.

- **Part(s) used**: bark

- **Preparation**: Brew this herb into tea or use its tincture with beverages and other edibles. Apply the ointment topically.

- **Recommended dosage**: 240 to 480 mg daily

- **Application methods**: There are several ways to take this herb. You can drink the tincture or add it to a beverage. You can also steep the dried version in hot water or brew tea with it.

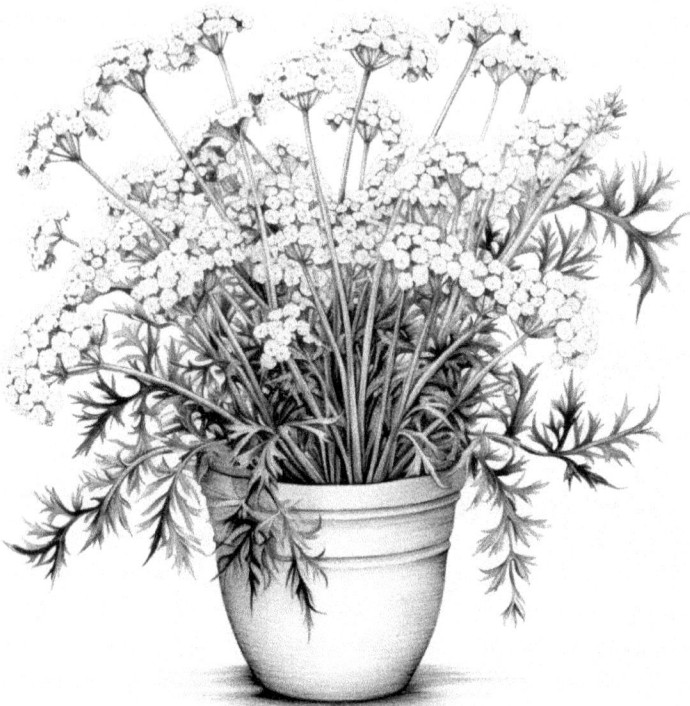

Yarrow

- **Healing applications**: Yarrow promotes faster wound recovery, lowers body temperature, eases digestive discomfort, reduces inflammation, addresses menstrual cramps, supports respiratory health, may help manage hypertension, assists in fluid balance, alleviates tension headaches, is used for stomach problems, may reduce allergy symptoms, calms nervousness, and anxiety, is a topical application for skin issues, eases arthritis discomfort, and supports cardiovascular health.

- **Side effects**: Some potential adverse reactions to this herb are sensitivity to sunlight and skin irritation.

- **Native habitat**: It originated in Europe and Asia and grows in many states, including California, Oregon, Washington, Montana, Idaho, Wyoming, Colorado, Utah, Arizona, New Mexico, Texas, Alaska, and more.

- **Part(s) used**: leaves, flowers, and stems

- **Preparation**: teas, tinctures, extracts, capsules, oils, and powders

- **Recommended dosage**: unknown

- **Application methods**: There are several ways to take this herb. You can drink the tincture or add it to a beverage. You can also steep the dried version in hot water or brew tea with it. The oil is normally used topically.

Conclusion

America has over 1000 medicinal herbs that are currently grown in various states. It's my ambition to provide detailed and accurate information on all these herbs to help many people reduce their dependence on big pharma and be medically prepared for any future disasters. A section of my website is dedicated to medicinal herbs for that purpose. You can subscribe for free on the website to get a notification whenever I publish new lists of herbs and related articles.

In the next chapter, I'll teach you how to obtain any herb, whether online or by foraging or gardening. You'll also learn about preparing all the concoctions I kept mentioning in the current chapter and how to store them in an apothecary you'll use now and later. You need to get active in preparing these local drugs, even if you won't use them now, so you can perfect the skill to the point where you won't need help or a guide formulating herbal remedies.

Chapter 4:

Herbal Prepping—the Tools and Techniques You Need From Nature

The doctor of the future will give no medication but will instruct his patient in the care of the human frame, in diet and in the cause and prevention of disease. –**Thomas Edison**

Now that you've seen a relatively large number of medicinal herbs and their uses, it's time to learn how to obtain these herbs, prepare them, build an apothecary and natural first aid, and grow an herbal garden. Acquiring some herbs promptly might be on your agenda. Let's begin with the most straightforward approach: purchasing them.

How to Buy the Right Herbs

If you want to buy herbs, you can get them from individuals and companies alike. Both can give you organic and genetically modified organism (GMO) herbs, depending on what you want. Even if you own a big garden, online sellers will sometimes help you gain access to herbs that aren't in your garden when you need them. Online shops are great sources of quality dried herbs, but you must choose wisely not to end up with faded, dusty, stale, or old herbs. Herbal products for sale can be found in many places, not just online. Grocery stores, local nurseries, and farmers markets are alternative places to get them (Karen, 2020). Here are the factors to consider when buying herbs online or in person:

- non-GMO certifications

- purity certification

- method of processing

- how an herb is packaged

- storage condition and duration

- seller's reputation

Non-GMO Certifications

The genetic combination of a herb is what gives it the ability to fight certain diseases in humans. A herb may have genes that allow it to produce high amounts of allicin, a highly beneficial plant compound with strong antibacterial properties. If this gene is altered in any way, it may result in higher or lower amounts of allicin or a less potent or more potent allicin. But what really happens to GMO herbs?

What it Means for an Herb to be GMO

Genetically modified organisms (plants and animals) have had their natural genetic combinations altered. Herbal companies can modify the genetic makeup of certain plants for various reasons, including pest control, resistance to insecticides, higher yields, and more (Diaz & Fridovich-Keil, 2018). GMO practices occur at the molecular level. In a molecular-level modification, breeders introduce the genes of different plants into the particular plant they want to modify.

They do this using *recombinant DNA technology*. Plants like garlic are high in allicin, a compound known to be effective against multi-drug-resistant bacteria (Shang et al., 2019). An herbal company can genetically modify garlic plants to produce higher yields, control pests and diseases, or create resistance against certain herbicides. This is certain to alter some chemical characteristics of the plant in a way that increases or reduces its medicinal value, depending on what you want garlic for.

Why the Medicinal Value Changes

Some changes that may occur with the plant's compounds as it grows would be unforeseen or uncontrollable. This may undermine certain properties of the plant. In the case of garlic, it may result in less amounts of allicin or other desired compounds. Consequently, you won't derive as much antibacterial benefits from this GMO garlic as you would from natural species. Some genetic modifications completely wipe out certain plant characteristics. Not all genetic modifications are bad. If it still retains sufficient amounts of the compounds in which you are interested, there's nothing wrong with using a GMO herb.

Natural Modifications Are Acceptable

Other ways herbal companies can grow desired plant breeds are through reproductive cloning and selective breeding. With reproductive cloning, companies try to grow herbs that are genetically identical to a parent plant. This parent plant may or may not be GMO. Selective breeding on the other hand is the practice of isolating individual plants from a group and growing them separately. This is done because of their superior qualities although they have the same genetic makeup as their inferior siblings.

If both selective breeding and reproductive cloning are done from non-GMO plants, then you may have a natural herb with potentially extraordinary qualities. Selective breeding and reproductive cloning are totally fine because no changes occur at the molecular level of the plant, which means its properties remain intact.

How to Verify an Herb's Naturality

You should request certification from companies that can afford them. Third-party testing costs money in most cases, and small or local farmers usually cannot afford that luxury. Asking them is the best way to confirm the nature of their herbs. Some would like to have you buy. The Organic Integrity Database is a useful tool for locating herbal companies whose plants are non-GMO. You can search the database by State, city, country, and other refinements.

You can also find out about how a herb was grown by asking locals, doing online research, visiting their farms, or even testing a sample if you can. We are talking about establishing long-term relationships here, so the extra work of verifying naturality is worth it. Always request proof of naturality from companies and other large businesses because they have no logical excuse for not being certified, except that perhaps they didn't or won't pass it.

Purity Certification of Herbal Products

Herbs growing on soil contaminated with heavy metals or pesticide residue may pose significant health risks to humans. Heavy metals like zinc, cadmium, copper, and lead are known to cause a range of diseases including lung cancer, cardiac failure, osteoporosis, renal dysfunction, and more. Pesticides can cause hormonal changes, hypersensitivity, asthma, and cancer (Alengebawy et al., 2021). You don't want to trigger any of these problems while trying to treat others. This risk is very high with geophytes, that is, plants with underground storage organs, such as bulbs, rhizomes, tubers, corms, and others.

So, if you are buying geophyte herbs, ensure they are free of heavy metals and pesticides, and if in doubt, wash them thoroughly or peel the skin to get rid of any impurities. However, some impurities are taken up by plants, which makes them difficult or even impossible to remove. The safest option is to buy herbs grown in, not on healthy soil. Request certifications against impurities from any seller or company eager to sell you herbs.

Herbal plants also should not be grown with fertilizers because they usually impact the herb's chemical composition. For example, fertilizers tend to reduce the vitamin C content of plants (Better Health, 2012). Some producers also use chemical additives to flavor their herbal products or extend their shelf lives. Insist on seeing their certification if you don't like any of them. You'll ingest a good dose of fertilizer chemicals if you buy herbs grown with them, particularly when using any parts other than fruits. One common excuse you'd receive from producers is that their formula is a proprietary blend. This implies that they cannot disclose significant details about the manufacturing process. Don't buy that.

Method of Processing

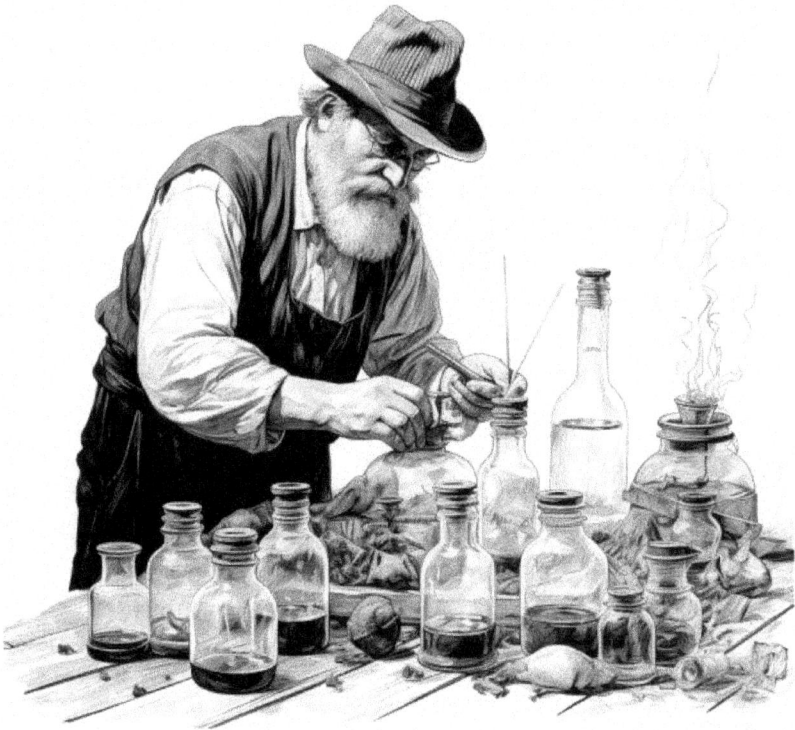

A herb's compounds start to degrade from the moment the plant is harvested and continue to deteriorate as the herb passes through various processes before reaching you. Any consumer wants an herb to be as close to its original state as possible when they receive the package.

Chemical changes occur in an herb while it's being processed. The extent of these changes depends on the processes applied to the plant. Drying, heating, pasteurizing, and even packaging cause significant alterations to an herb's constituents. You deserve to know what processes an herb passes through to get a good idea of the likely concentration of any compounds or ingredients you are interested in. Some companies disclose the preparatory steps of their herbal remedies while others hide behind manufacturing secrets or other excuses to avoid full disclosure.

Why Processing Is Important

Water-soluble vitamins easily break down while processing plants, especially during processes that involve heat. But nutrient loss doesn't happen at the same rate for all kinds of heating. For example, microwave cooking supersedes boiling and destroying vitamin K, while boiling destroys more vitamin C than microwave cooking does (Lee et al., 2017). Therefore, if you want an herbal product with high quantities of certain compounds for your health needs, try to find out what processing methods destroy such compounds and to what extent.

Ask the company about their manufacturing methods. If it's likely to destroy your preferred compounds, it's better to explore other options. For example, let's assume you are looking for a specific herb that is very high in vitamin C, and you come across a supplier who pasteurized or sterilized herbs before packaging them. We know that pasteurizing is one of the industrial processes that degrade vitamin C. As such, you shouldn't buy the herb from this dealer due to the high risk of getting low-quality stuff.

How an Herb Is Packaged

Some plant ingredients are sensitive to light, air, and moisture. All three can degrade the plant's natural constituents. Packaging that doesn't effectively block them results in low shelf life and lower-quality products. If you want to buy an herb whose ingredients are vulnerable to light, ensure that the packaging effectively blocks light from penetrating the container. You don't know how long it had been in storage before your purchase. Packaging with opaque or colored plastic works well for such herbs.

Vitamin C is sensitive to light, and if you are buying an herb for its high vitamin C content, the package seal must be light-proof. A quick Google search can usually confirm that. Additionally, you shouldn't buy fresh herbs from a seller who doesn't use breathable material for packaging. Fresh herbs need airy containers to prevent rotting, especially during shipping when the package may be exposed to light or heat.

Storage Condition and Duration

The potency of an herb doesn't improve in storage and can only deteriorate rapidly or slowly depending on its environment. The most important elements that affect herbs in storage include light, time, ambient aroma, humidity, and temperature. Herbs stored for a long time aren't as potent as fresh or more recent ones. You want to know how long an herb has been in storage before buying it. It's more common to find old herbs in grocery stores than online. But still, you need to be careful with online purchases because some suppliers would rather ship out old stock than make losses (EHA Consulting Group, n.d.).

Seller Reputation

The field of herbal medicine isn't regulated by the government. Therefore, quality control is still weak or even nonexistent in the US. The burden of verifying quality is on your shoulders. Thankfully, there are third-party organizations and institutions certifying companies and individuals dealing with herbs, though these certifications are voluntary. Certified sellers are more reliable when it comes to quality.

Make sure the seller knows a lot about herbs before patronizing them. The herbal industry is full of amateur sellers—maybe because it's still young and growing. Amateurs are more likely to make mistakes in deliveries. Some plants can be mislabeled or incorrectly identified by the producer, which won't solve your problem and may even cause health problems (Noveille, 2021b).

Foraging for Wild Herbs

The first thing to take care of when foraging for herbs is your physical safety. This pertains to your safety in the wild and from the herbs you've harvested for consumption. The second most important thing is the legal aspect of foraging. It's legal to harvest herbs and fungi on any government-owned land. Let's start with your physical safety and divide it into three parts:

- What not to collect in the wild

- What you wear and carry

- How you forage

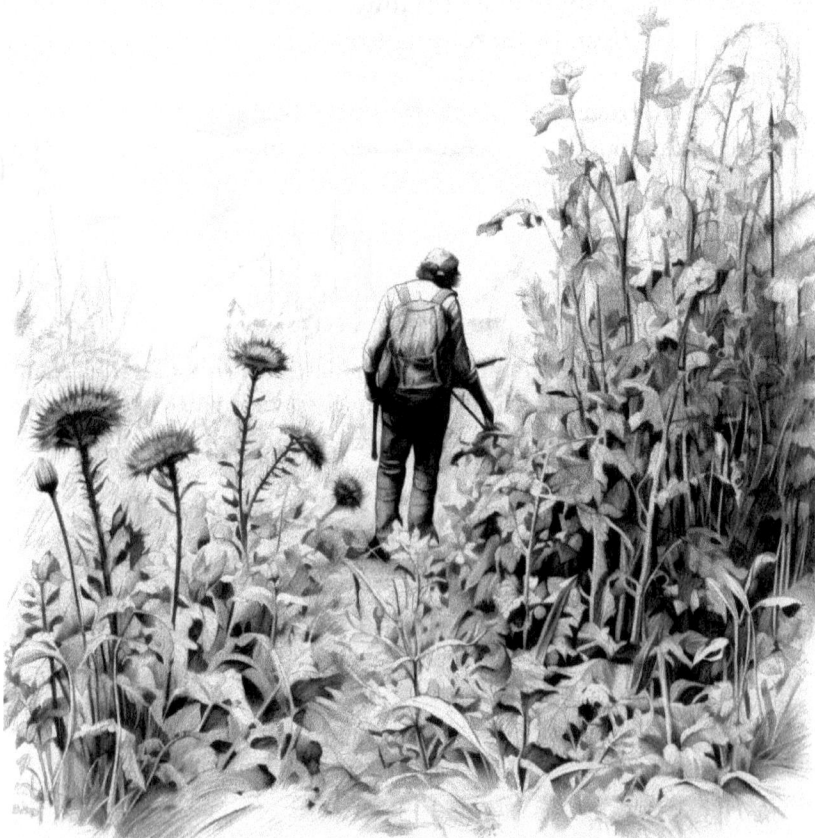

What Not to Collect in the Wild

In the world of herbal prepping, picking wild herbs shows our deep connection to nature. Exploring the wild uncovers plants with healing and cooking uses, each telling its own story. This chapter shares how best to forage for wild herbs, from picking the right plants to avoiding certain elements to using the proper tools. It's more than just botany—it's about respecting nature. This guide covers everything, focusing on safety in the wild to keep both nature and foragers safe.

It's advantageous to compile a list of desired herbs and their necessary quantities before venturing into the wild. This practice minimizes the time spent foraging and prevents your bag from being filled with lower-priority herbs. A detailed list would direct your exercise to the right type and quantity of herbs. It'll also prevent you from picking the wrong plants or collecting more than you need.

Be Wary of Places Open to Animals

Domestic and wild animals can carry dangerous pathogens that are harmless to them but deadly to humans. Foxes, birds, rats, and dogs are skilled at infiltrating spaces in search of sustenance or simply to wander. Their instincts prompt them to urinate and defecate wherever the need arises, disseminating waste filled with potentially harmful substances and organisms. This is why you must be careful where to plug herbs and use those herbs. Plants growing closer to the ground are less safe than their taller siblings. That's because they are more likely to collect urine, feces, and other badass substances. But this doesn't imply that tall plants are safe to consume without washing or sterilizing.

Foraging plant leaves or fruits in areas frequented by wild or domestic birds poses a risk of Salmonella contamination. Bird droppings may contain this bacterium, transferring it to vegetation through contact. Consumption of contaminated plants can lead to Salmonella infection in humans, causing gastrointestinal distress and other health complications. Proper hygiene, thorough washing of foraged produce, and avoiding areas heavily populated by birds mitigate this risk during foraging activities.

237

Scrutinize Plants for Health Issues

Before embarking on your herb-gathering quest, familiarize yourself with what a healthy specimen looks like. Various indicators can reveal if a plant is encountering any issues or struggles. Some of the signs include changing leaf color, wilting leaves, leaves dotted black, drooping leaves, brown leaf edges, yellowing leaves, visible roots, leaves with yellow rings around brown marks, yellow leaves, poor flower development, unnatural spots, and changing leaf colors (Canaway, 2019). If a plant doesn't look healthy to you, especially when compared to identical species, it probably isn't.

The fact that a plant is looking very green, fresh, and healthy doesn't mean it's safe to take. Maybe it's growing in a convenient spot, such as at the base of trees or nearby shrubs. These are places where people are more inclined to urinate. Some urine may touch the leaves and even penetrate their pores. Urine is everything your kidney considers toxic to the body. By consuming items contaminated by urine, you risk developing kidney disease and organ damage as your system works harder to deal with an increased concentration of toxic substances in the body.

Avoid Places Exposed to Pollution

Pollution is the primary reason why foraging in cities isn't a good idea. Gaseous, liquid, and solid wastes can all contaminate plants. Particulates of soot, dust, and smoke from machines can accumulate on plant leaves and stems, hindering normal growth and development. Plant leaves have invisible holes in them called the stomata through which transpiration occurs. Some particulates can penetrate the stomata and remain stuck in there no matter how rigorously you wash the herb.

This is why you should be very wary of foraging within the city or by roadsides. Pesticides, herbicides, and other chemicals can wholly contaminate a plant from the flowers down to the roots. We learned in Chapter Two that these chemicals can cause serious health issues in people. Only forage in built-up areas, if you are confident the plants have not been exposed to any pollutants, like when they are far from roads and the area, isn't subject to herbicide or pesticide use.

Look Out for Poisonous Plants

Pick herbs carefully because some grow together with dangerous plants that are poisonous when ingested. Don't allow unwanted plants in your collections unless you are sure they are harmless. Remove any plants you don't know or identify as harmful.

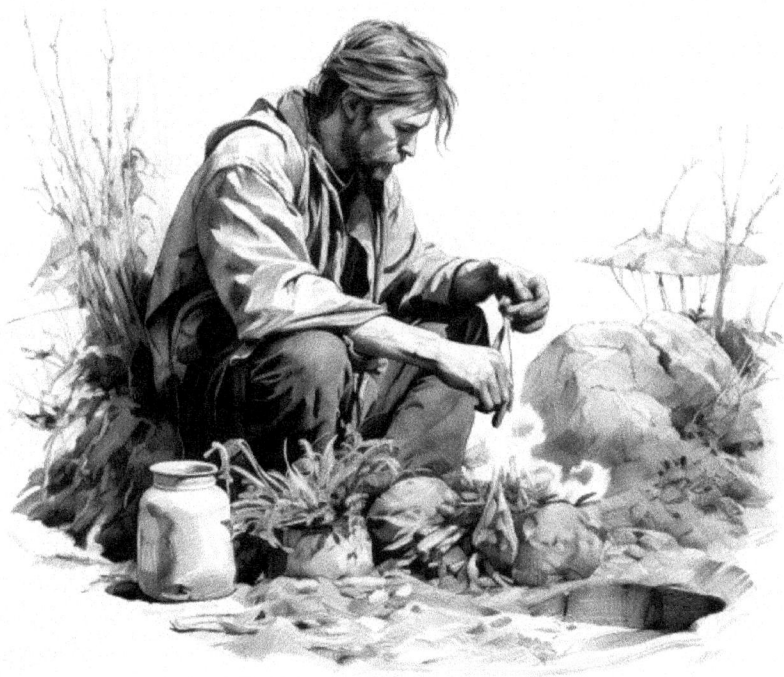

What You Wear and Carry

Wild environments demand attire different from your everyday wear. Unlike your work environment, the wild requires specialized clothing for confidence, comfort, and safety during foraging. Within this section, we'll detail various essential items to enhance your foraging experience.

The Clothes to Put On

Wear breathable clothes because your trip into the wild may last hours depending on how fast you find the herbs. Prepare for the long haul to be on the safe side. In addition to breathable clothes, put on sweat-wicking underwear that keeps your skin dry. You may consider wearing a lightweight jacket that insulates your body from the cold. If foraging in the rainy season or the weather looks kind of rainy, a rain jacket may be necessary as an outer layer.

Ensure that your clothing is durable and protects from scratches, insect bites, piercings, abrasions, and plant hairs (trichomes) that may cause rashes or itching. Many plants cause discomfort when they contact your skin, such as Poison Ivy, Poison Oak, Poison Sumac, Wood Nettle, Stinging Nettle, Baby's Breath, Leadwort, and more (Strauch, 2022).

Protecting Your Feet and Hands

You need a pair of boots that are sturdy, closed-toed, with good ankle support and a strong grip on the ground for navigating uneven and slippery terrains. Hiking boots are the most appropriate for foraging. A pair of moisture-absorbing socks that will protect from blisters by keeping the feet dry. I also suggest you slap on a wide-brimmed hat and wear sunglasses for protection from the sun, insects, and tiny objects. Depending on the kind of animals living where you intend to forage, a camouflage outfit may offer extra protection by blending you in with the surroundings and making you difficult to spot by wild animals (Gravalese, 2023). A pair of trichome-proof hand gloves should protect your hands as you pick herbs.

How You Forage and What to Take Along

It's advisable to avoid foraging alone, even in less remote areas. Having company is beneficial—a second set of eyes may spot treasures you overlooked and can catch dangers like snakes or wild animals you might miss. Additionally, if you encounter a minor or major accident, having someone with you can be crucial, as handling it alone might be tough or even impossible. A companion is good anytime you forage because even if they don't have the competence to deal with an emergency, they can assist in finding help. Consider carrying a defensive weapon such as a gun or pepper spray in case you encounter a dangerous animal or some bad guy out there, especially if you are foraging alone.

Always look before you leap. Dense vegetation can conceal various dangers, from snakes to insects, holes, cliffs, quicksand, and more. When faced with thick vegetation, survey a herb's environment critically before attempting to go in. Your attire and tools may not provide adequate protection from some unfriendly environments and creatures.

Get all the Tools You Need

For the best foraging experience, you need to have all the necessary tools, including:

- bag

- basket

- shears

- knife

- small nylon bags

- sickle

- mini garden tools

- tiny rubber bands

The Bag

Staying longer in the wilderness becomes possible when you haven't gathered all the necessary herbs in time. The initial plants you collect remain stored in your bag for the duration of your journey. Leaves and flowers, when enclosed, can degrade in medicinal properties swiftly due to heat. A well-ventilated bag reduces temperature, preserving the effectiveness of your medicines (*The Forager's Toolkit*, 2020).

The Basket

For picking flowers, a basket will save you a lot of trouble. Perhaps the flowers have pollen you want to take home. If this pollen scatters in a bag, collecting it won't be easy since it may dust everything in there. This is why you should take a basket along when targeting flowers. It's important to line the basket with newspapers to prevent pollen from dusting off through the holes. Additionally, flowers are pretty vulnerable to heat and won't endure for long in a closed bag.

The Knife

The knife should be stainless steel because you'll use it on dewy plants too. It should be convenient to use, sturdy, and sharp. The knife will be your most frequently used tool as it's applicable in a range of tasks, including cutting, chopping, slicing, batoning, and more. Even if you don't perform some of these in the wild, you may do them upon returning home. Avoid knives with very narrow or wide blades unless they are suited to certain tasks you want to accomplish (Law, 2023).

shears

This is a critical foraging tool. Using a flat or curved knife to cut specific plant parts is simply impractical and time-consuming. Branches and stems can be malleable, meaning they don't snap when you try to break them. These are harder to cut with a knife than shears. With shears, you just gather and snip. You can conveniently cut finger-sized stems with this tool.

Nylon Bags

Nylon bags are important for organizing different plant roots and seeds. You'll avoid mixing up the roots and soiling your bag's interior with dirt.

If you come across fruits, dumping them together with leaves and roots isn't a good idea. It's also impractical to tie fruits together with rubber bands. Plant roots you dig up will have random lengths that make bundling with rubber bands clumsy or even impractical. Seeds should be separated from leaves and roots as well.

The Sickle

The sickle is the best tool for harvesting grassy herbs. You can fetch a large bundle in a single cut. The historical function of a sickle is to collect forage for animals and harvest grains. It lets you gather a large pile of grassy herbs in no time. However, it must be sharp and sturdy for convenient foraging. The handles should be smooth and have good friction. A large sickle isn't necessary for foraging since you won't be collecting huge grass piles.

Mini Gardening Tools

Gardening equipment can work for foraging but most can't fit in a bag and are clumsy or heavy to slug around. They include a spade, hoe, scraper, looper, axe, pickaxe and more. However, the mini versions of these tools are available online. I particularly like the scraper and shovel for digging up plant roots. These two also fit easily into a bag.

Tiny Rubber Bands

Tiny rubber bands are a must-have for collecting leafy or grassy herbs. Dumping various leaves together in a bag creates the extra work of separating them when you return home. Others will remain in the wrong collection even after careful separation. Rubber bands also prevent leaves from scattering and taking up more space, though with the advantage of allowing more ventilation.

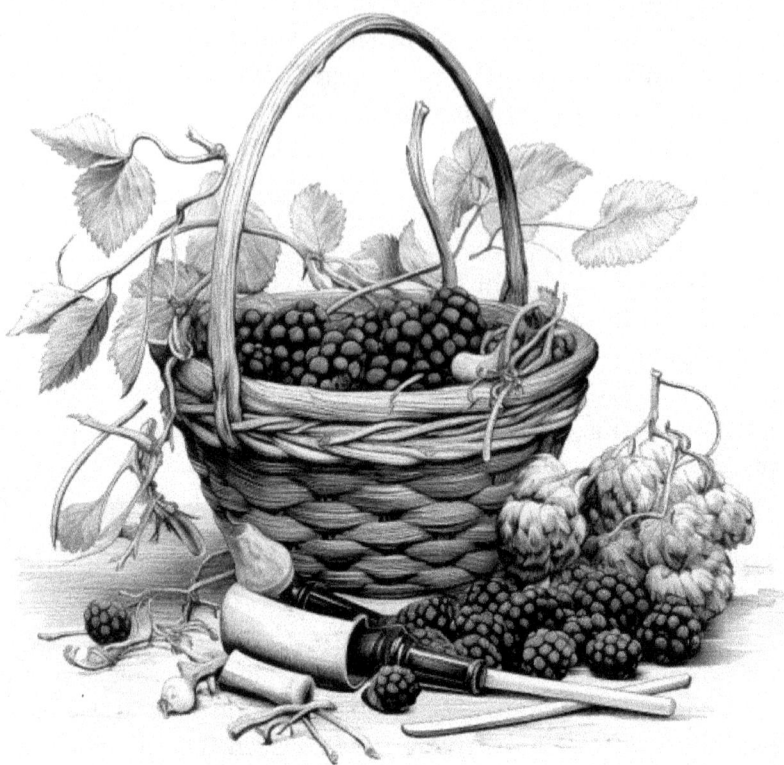

Forage Responsibly

Resist the temptation to exhaustively harvest discovered herbs or edibles, especially rare varieties, unless you can genuinely utilize the entire yield—a rarity due to shelf life and dosage limitations. It's essential to forage responsibly, avoiding needless destruction of plants others could benefit from. While it's not mandatory to leave behind herbs if your harvest falls short, erring on the side of caution is imprudent. Overharvesting could deprive others of the same resource. Returning for more is wiser than taking excess; it ensures sustainability and the availability of resources for all (Institute of Culinary Education, 2018).

Try to avoid foraging on private properties because it can lead to legal problems. Some landowners may suspect you are more than foraging. Another legal obstacle to foraging is *protected plant species*. We know that thousands of plants are endangered, and the government may have imposed restrictions on harvesting some of them. When possible, do advanced research on endangered species in your foraging location to steer clear of any troubles.

Pro Tip on Foraging: "Correctly" identify all the plants within foraging distance and map out their medicinal uses, especially the abundant varieties. Google is your best buddy for this task. These are the plants you can always have access to during emergencies. Exploit the medicinal uses of the plants around you before looking beyond. Some can be good substitutes for unavailable species.

Starting an Herbal Garden From Scratch

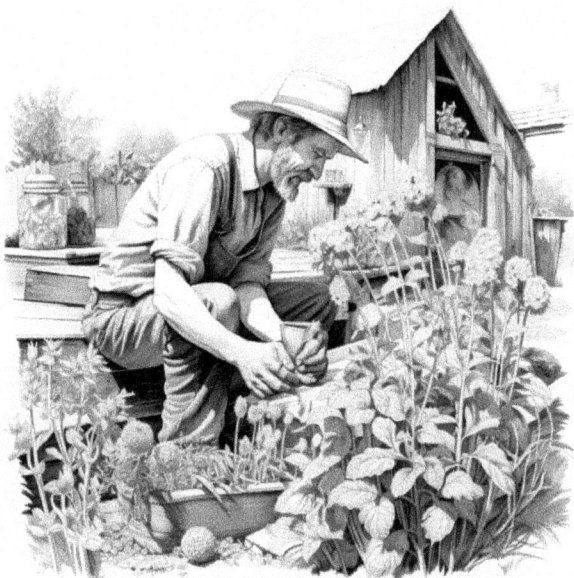

Frequently, there might not be both the funds and time available to purchase or gather herbs, especially for consistent users. Moreover, both buying and foraging come with drawbacks, notably the uncertainty surrounding their quality and safety. Regularly using fresh herbs is difficult when you rely on vendors and foraging. Most times, the leaves wilt before reaching your pot or blender.

The most reliable way to obtain the herbs you want is to farm them. Herbal gardening is a rewarding activity that can produce valuable greens, support many people, generate income, and give you total control over the quantity and quality of herbs to use. It can also offer great leeway over diseases and your family's health. Working in a garden exerts a calming effect on the mind, which is another form of promoting health.

Those who want a transition to herbal medicine will enjoy doing that with an herbal garden for support. Imagine the confidence and peace of mind of knowing all the medicine you need is just a few minutes away. Your herbal garden is a form of the natural apothecary—It's a green and sustainable pharmacy. Here are the steps for starting a herbal garden from the ground up:

1. research the herbs to plant

2. choose a favorable location

3. decide on a garden-type

4. map out territory by species

5. test the Soil

6. prepare the soil for cultivation

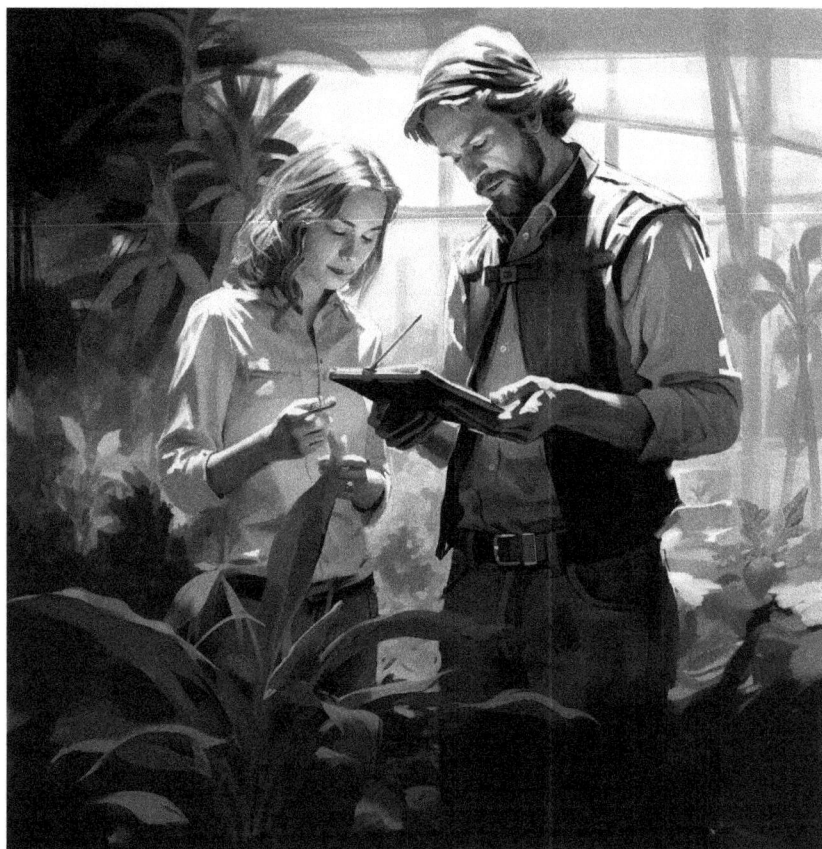

Research the Herbs to Plant

From your current and potential future health challenges, choose herbs that will solve your problems and then research them to know whether they can survive the local climate. Also, find out how easy it is to obtain the seeds and the planting methods. Other important information includes the average mature size, sunlight and water requirements, the necessary nutrients, and soil condition.

Choose a Favorable Location

Designate a location before sourcing seeds or nurseries to plant. This is important because locations can have full or partial exposure to the sun and some herbs need more sunlight than others. You'll know from the plot's landscaping whether certain herbs will do well on it. Plant them where the sun shines most during the day. It's while graphing the garden that plant positioning is implemented.

Decide on a Garden-Type

What type of garden do you want to plant? Will you plant the seeds in the ground, garden pots, or above-ground containers? Choose a garden type and size you can manage because it's a long-term affair. Grooming plants to maturity can be tough, particularly in the early stages when they are delicate and need greater care. Gardening is most enjoyable in your backyard, but if you lack open land, a balcony or patio can serve just as well.

Map Out Territory by Species

You'll be planting different herbs in the same garden. Identify the areas receiving the most sunlight in order to plant corresponding herbs there. Some herbs need more sunlight than others. Don't situate them in shadowy areas if there are species more tolerant of shade. Certain shrubby herbs, such as elderberries, spirea, ninebark, and others, can grow anywhere with little sunlight a day (Coulter & Forney, n.d.). So, do not misplace priority when planting your herbs.

Test the Soil

The test results determine the necessity and extent of soil improvement. For the optimal growth of medicinal herbs, soil nutrients play a pivotal role. These plants thrive in soils rich in essential nutrients such as nitrogen, phosphorus, potassium, and various organic matter. Nitrogen aids in robust foliage development, while phosphorus supports root growth and overall plant vitality.

Potassium contributes to disease resistance and enhances the herb's essential oil production. Additionally, organic matter enriches the soil structure, fostering microbial activity crucial for nutrient absorption by the herbs. The balance and richness of these nutrients in the soil are fundamental for cultivating robust and potent medicinal herbs. Testing the soil before planting is crucial to assess its nutrient composition and pH levels for an optimal growing environment.

Prepare the Garden for Planting

Prepare your plot by clearing it and breaking up the soil, making it easier to create smooth rows or ridges in your garden. Ridges should be 6–8 inches tall to ease planting, and about 4 feet wide to provide irrigation access to all plants (CropWatch, 2015). Leave enough walkways between ridges, about 24 inches, so you can conveniently manage the garden (*A Guide to Fruit and Vegetable*, n.d.).

You'll be spacing the herbs while graphing your garden. Proper spacing gives plants room for full growth. It lets them spread roots and branches as far as possible for optimal development. The herbs won't tangle up their branches, and this makes harvesting and weed control easier. To know how much space an herb needs, figure out its average mature size. This information is usually available on plant tags and catalogs. For example, if the herb grows to five feet wide, measure five feet from the stem, round. That's how much space a plant needs for uninterrupted growth and development. Every herb should have sufficient growth space according to its average maturity size (Toscano, 2022).

Managing Weeds in the Garden

Plan weed control beforehand so you won't regret it if weeding proves a mighty challenge later. It may be in your best interest to use landscape fabric or geotextile for weed control. Geotextile prevents weeds from growing in the first place. It's a carpet-like material that is laid a few inches beneath the topsoil. Water, air, nutrients, and plant roots can easily penetrate through, but weeds are barred. Geotextile costs money but is indispensable for people who cannot or do not want to control weeds. Once decided on weed control, it's time to plant.

Conclusion

This chapter explains how anyone can obtain herbs. It emphasized three options including buying, foraging, and gardening. My advice is for you to start purchasing herbs online or locally before foraging or building a garden. The reason is that you'll learn a lot from vendors and you'll experience many herbs before foraging or growing them. The herbs your body accepts without serious allergies should be priority number one if or when you venture into the wild to collect medicine.

Foraging is important because not only will you get the herbs for free but you will also get the quantities you want. The main disadvantage of foraging is that you may come back without some critical herbs you desire. Additionally, there are safety risks in terms of quality and your well-being. But I've explained the measures to be taken to minimize the chances of any unpleasant events.

Gardening is the most reliable and easy way to obtain quality herbs. You are in control of what grows in the garden and who accesses it. If you want to seriously try herbs in your life, I recommend starting an organic garden. You can set it some distance from home in the absence of a nearby gardening space.

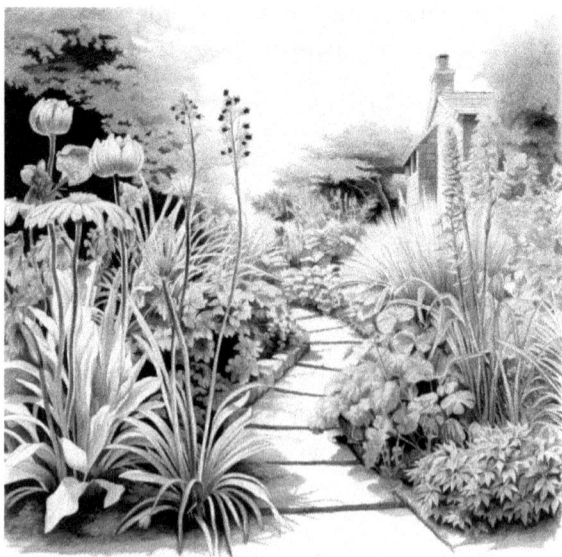

Chapter 5:

Natural Healing Solutions—

Building Your Green Pharmacy

The greatest gift you can give your family and the world is a healthy you. –Joyce Meyer

This chapter is about the skills for making herbal remedies, building an apothecary and natural first aid, and adopting the holistic philosophy of herbalism. It explains skills that will help you to create, store, and use herbal medicines. Literally, you'll become an herbalist and be able to commercialize your expertise and herbal collections as you wish.

It would be best if you learned to create different herbal remedies, from tinctures to salves and medicated bar soaps. It's possible to degrade the potency of an herb by how it's made. That's why you must pay close attention while formulating any remedies. I'll list the most important forms of herbal remedies you should learn to prepare and briefly describe how to make them. Then, we'll see the proper way to build and organize an apothecary and a natural first aid kit. We'll conclude with some basics on the principles and philosophies for optimal benefit from herbalism. Let's jump in.

Formulating Medicines From Herbs

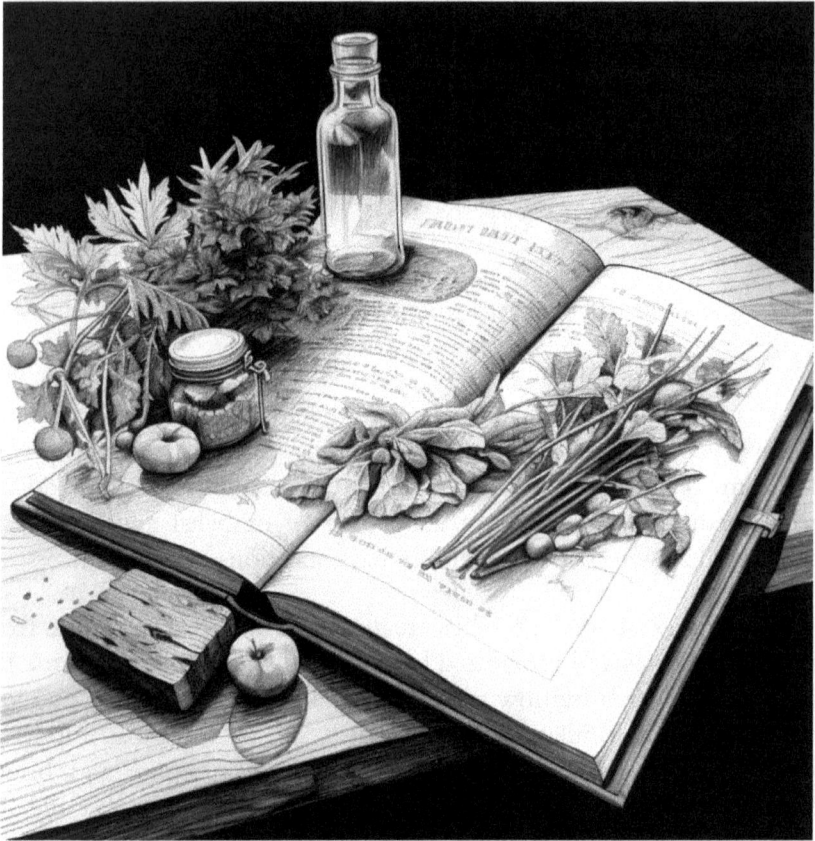

During emergencies, diverse herbal applications might be necessary. Health issues could call for ingestion of remedies, topical application on wounds or the body, or the use of eye and ear drops. Certain herbs prove beneficial for oral care or as part of therapeutic baths for skin ailments. A well-prepared herbal first aid kit and apothecary should encompass remedies for managing bleeding and alleviating pain resulting from insect bites, burns, swellings, fractures, dislocations, and a range of other ailments.

If you're adept at crafting remedies for various health challenges and have access to the necessary raw materials, you possess the skills of a proficient herbalist capable of addressing health crises during disasters.

Moreover, this valuable expertise can be monetized during peaceful times. Let's examine these concoctions one by one and classify them by mode of use.

Herbal Remedies Used Internally

Most herbal formulas are for internal use. Herbs that are safe for ingestion can be taken in liquid or solid forms. However, the fear and inconvenience of taking medicine forces herbalists to innovate forms that are easy and pleasing to ingest. As an example, edible herbs can be converted into soap-like solids. But this form won't be convenient to use. Similarly, a solidified herbal cream will be a burden to use. The same logic applies to watery herbal soaps. All the exemplified formations are usable but with serious inconveniences.

Back to the internal use of herbs.

The best herbal forms for internal use include tinctures, capsules, teas, juices, recipes, gels, tablets, gums, syrups, powder, teas, and oils, among others. We'll see how to transform the flowers, leaves, stems, etc., harvested into easy-to-consume concoctions.

Herbal Remedies Used Externally

External-use Herbal forms can be solids (soaps), tinctures (ear or eye drops), powders, gels, essential oils, pastes, and creams. The challenge for most herbalists is how to convert plant ingredients into these forms. Obviously, no amount of heating can change tinctures into gels or powders into gums. There's a need for natural or plant-based additives that won't interfere with the medicinal functions of the herb or its convenient use. Let's discuss the raw materials used for transforming herbal extracts into any form, liquid, solid, or gas. You must know how to make or obtain these raw materials to be a fully independent herbalist. Here are the most important ones:

- essential oil

- honey, wax, and gum

- soap

- gels

- alcohol and vinegar

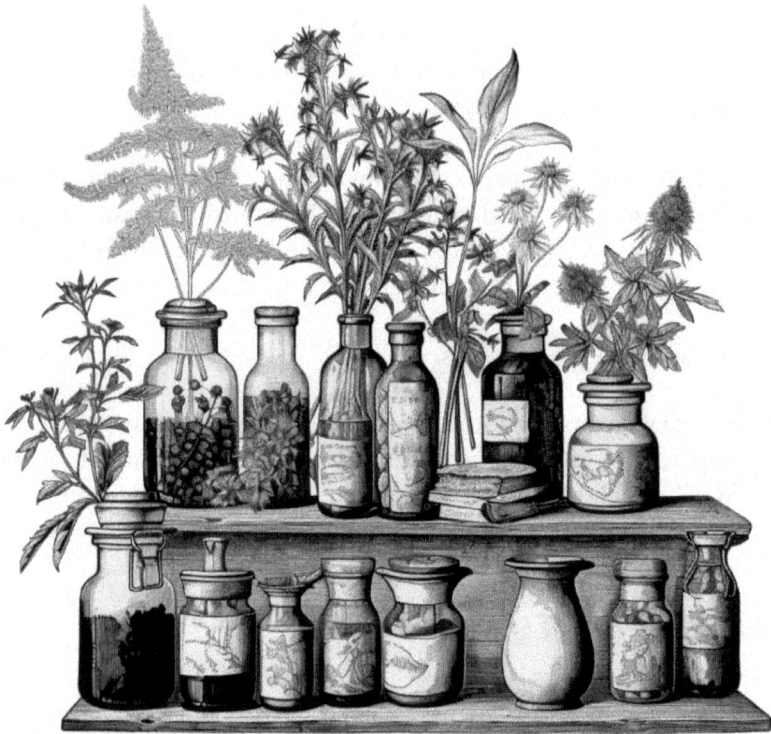

Essential Oils

There are several ways to extract essential oil from biomass (materials from plants and animals). Plant biomass includes seeds, roots, leaves, fruit peels, flowers, and others. This mass of organic matter can contain lots of trapped oil you can extract by distillation, cold compress, solvent extraction, and CO_2 extraction (Klinger, 2021).

Honey, Wax, and Gum

Beekeeping is one of the easiest activities for herbalists and preppers. You can do this in your backyard. Just build or purchase a beehive; buy some bee swarms or nuclear colonies from any nearby apiary. There are different types of beehives; a little research will quickly point you in the right direction to buy the one most appealing and convenient for you. The Langstroth beehive is very popular in America as it's very practical with an attractive design (Garman, 2019).

Soaps

In many African traditions, soap is made from plant alkali and palm kernel oil. Any plant biomass that produces sufficient amounts of potassium after combustion can be used to produce the alkali you need to make soap. Examples of such biomass include sugar-beet chaff, plantain and banana peels, wood, cocoa pods, palm branches, maize cobs, and more. You can make an antiseptic soap from these ingredients if you add shea butter, honey, or coconut oil to the mix. The process produces top-quality soap with good foam if done properly. The ashes of these plant parts contain significant amounts of potassium, and when dissolved in distilled water and filtered, the ash solution can have a high concentration of potassium hydroxide (KOH). This is the solution you'll mix with any oil to produce soap, which you can further refine into solid bars (Igbashio, 2022).

To make soap, they gather biomass, dry and then burn it to ashes. The ash is mixed with water to form a thick paste and then dumped into a container with small holes at the bottom, like those of a colander. They allow sufficient space above the layer of ash. A desired quantity of water is gradually poured over the ash and allowed to drop through the small holes into another container. The filtrate, concentrated in KOH, may be slightly evaporated to increase the concentration before mixing it with palm kernel oil to make soap.

Gels

You can make gels from a range of plants, such as corn and cassava. This gel is safe to ingest and can be used to thicken your soaps, antibacterial tinctures, dental formulas, oils, and other herbal concoctions. The innermost parts of aloe vera leaves are good gel materials, especially if your formula is for external use (Alam, 2023).

Alcohol and Vinegar

Alcohol is better than water at extracting compounds from plants. But I'm not a fan of alcohol due to the health problems it can cause or exacerbate, such as liver disease. Any edible plant material that has sugar can be fermented into alcohol. If you extract the juice of such plants and mix in some bacteria or yeast, this will trigger a fermentation process where bacteria break down sugar into alcohol. Adding another acetic acid bacteria into the mix will gradually convert the alcoholic solution back into vinegar.

Vinegar requires alcoholic fermentation, followed by fermenting the alcoholic solution using acetic acid bacteria. The bacteria gradually reduces the alcoholic concentration to about 0.5% by converting it to acetic acid. This is why vinegar isn't alcoholic but acidic despite coming from alcohol. You can make vinegar from rice, apple cider, orange, corn, balsamic, and other sweet plants. In the next section, you'll read about herbal remedies that come from vinegar and alcohol.

What You Can Do With These Ingredients

Here are some of the herbal formulations achievable with the substances discussed above.

- herbal teas

- tinctures

- capsules

- salves

- poultices

- syrups and inhalations

Herbal Teas

You prepare herbal tea like you do normal tea. Boil water and drop in some dry leaves, powder, roots, and so on. You'd typically prepare this with a teapot or infuser, a cup, a sieve, and a spoon for stirring the mix. It takes 5–10 minutes for a tea to extract properly. You can add lemon or honey for flavor.

Tinctures

Tinctures are the resulting colored liquid obtained by soaking dried herbs in a solution for an extended period. This coloration represents the extraction of various compounds from the plant into the liquid, and contrary to expectation, water might not always be the primary solvent used in this process. Alcohol is better at extracting these compounds, but it can get you drunk and invite any of the problems alcohol is known to create. Vinegar is a safer and more effective way of extracting medicinal juices from dried herbs. Use a closed container for tincture and ensure everything stays submerged in the liquid. To speed up and make the process more complete, shake it daily and let it sit in a cool, dark place for 4–6 weeks.

Tinctures are concentrated liquid herbal extracts. Begin by filling a glass jar with 1 part dried herbs and 2 parts alcohol, such as vodka or brandy. Ensure the herbs are fully submerged. Seal the jar and place it in a cool, dark location for 4-6 weeks, shaking it daily to aid extraction. After the steeping period, strain the liquid, pressing the herbs to extract all the goodness. Store the resulting tincture in a tinted glass dropper bottle for easy dispensing. Hand-pressing the mix further draws out the compounds.

Capsules

If an herbal remedy is dried and you don't like the taste, capsules will disguise the unpleasant flavor. Grind it into fine powder with a grinder or mortar and pestle, and use a capsule-filling machine or your hands to fill the empty capsule shells you bought. You can also use capsules for herbs that require precise dosing, especially if you'll give it to someone.

Salves

Salves are solidified substances containing medicinal herbs. The only use of such oil is to convey the herb where you want, such as on the skin. You make salves by infusing dried herbs into oil and heating them over low heat for several hours so that the desired medicinal compounds spread into the oil. Mix it with beeswax to make a semi-solid mixture, which solidifies when placed in a container for some time.

Poultices

These are herbal pastes made by mixing crushed herbs with water. Aloe vera is one of the common herbs used to make poultices. The advantage of this herbal formation is that it doesn't dry quickly, which reduces the frequency of application.

Syrups and Inhalations

The syrup is essentially a blend of herbal tincture or infusion/tea combined with honey and reduced to a thick liquid consistency. Inhalations involve herbal remedies added to hot water, and you breathe in the resulting vapor. These remedies, in various forms, work as long as their vapor reaches your nose. For instance, inhaling chamomile flower essential oil vapor can alleviate feelings of depression or anxiety. Inhalations are herbal remedies you put in hot water and inhale the vapor. They can be in any form, provided their vapor reaches your nose. You can inhale the vapor of chamomile oil to ease depression or anxiety (Gupta, 2010).

You can make other concentrated extracts by infusing sufficient amounts of an herb in alcohol, vinegar, glycerine, carrier oil, and other solvents to condense and harmonize it. It is similar to herbal creams but thicker due to the beeswax.

Building an Herbal Apothecary

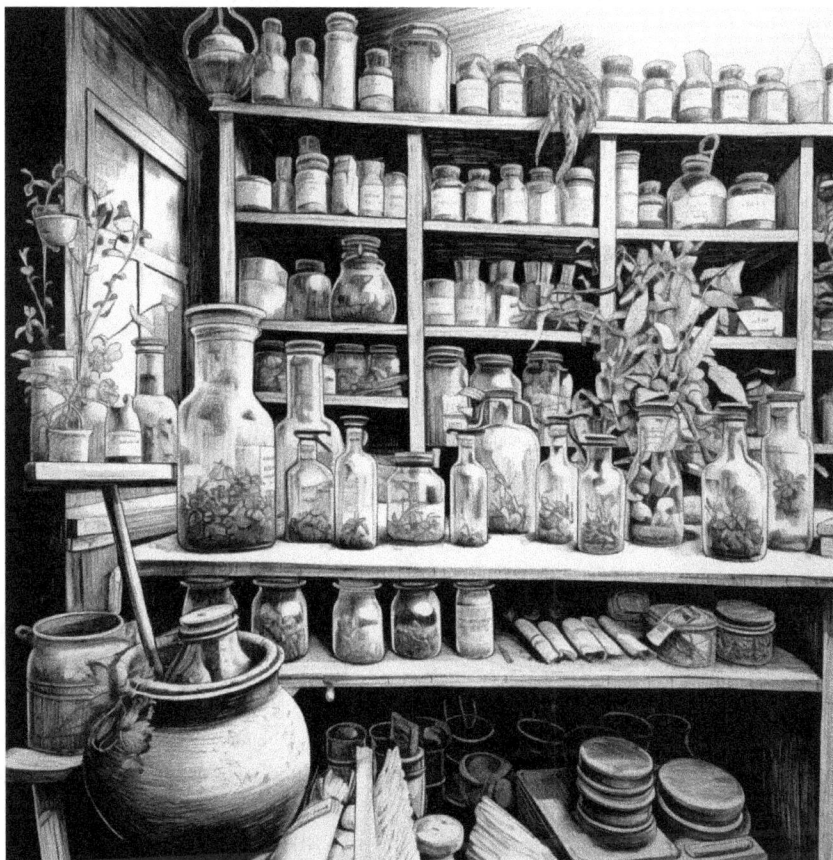

An herbal apothecary is a space or a collection of resources dedicated to storing, preparing, and utilizing herbal remedies and natural elements for health and wellness purposes. It typically includes a variety of dried herbs, tinctures, extracts, oils, and tools needed to create and administer herbal remedies. It serves as a hub for herbalists or individuals interested in natural healing, offering a wide range of herbs and materials to address various health concerns. Your green pharmacy should contain plant stems, roots, powders, tinctures, salves, and anything herbal. Avoid storing herbal remedies prone to quick spoilage in their finished forms within the apothecary. Instead, retain their entirety, like roots, stems, and similar parts.

The initial step in establishing an apothecary involves choosing the medicines to include. While many plants possess medicinal properties, their selection should align with specific needs. Filling the apothecary with unnecessary remedies serves little purpose unless they're intended for sale. Therefore, it's crucial to comprehend the criteria for selecting medicines that belong to an apothecary.

Consider four things when selecting apothecary collections.

- your current health status

- common sicknesses in your area

- most likely disasters for your town or city

- health challenges that typically come with such disasters

Your Current Health Status

You know your health better than anyone else. You also know the illnesses that have afflicted you in the past five or ten years. Your apothecary's first job is to free you of any illnesses and protect you against others. Make a list of all the health problems currently troubling you if they are known. Otherwise, you can go see your primary care physician for a full health checkup to get a better understanding of what health problems are lingering or are more likely to afflict you in the future. For example, some people have type 1 diabetes. It means they can possibly get Type 2.

Once you've identified your health concerns, begin researching herbs known for their healing and preventive properties related to those specific issues. Every plant medicine typically has substitutes. This means that for a particular ailment, there are often multiple plants that offer remedies, much like a single herb can address various diseases. If a specific herb isn't available in your area, seek out local alternatives that offer similar medicinal properties. Opt for plants that won't give you problems like allergies or worsened health conditions. If you consume certain foods or substances with potential health risks, find out the diseases they can cause and make sure the curative herbs are in your green pharmacy.

Common Diseases in Your Community

If you come across a community where many individuals are grappling with a specific illness, take caution and prepare yourself to avoid falling victim, particularly if you reside there or plan to do so. The same verdict goes for sicknesses that afflict most of the global population. In a community where many are affected by a certain ailment, it's wise to take precautions against it, even if you're not currently experiencing it yourself. Weather and environmental factors can impact various illnesses; for instance, warmer temperatures can exacerbate air quality issues and the spread of respiratory conditions. Being aware of these connections allows for proactive steps to protect your health, regardless of the specific climate (*Climate Impacts on Human Health*, n.d.).

Potential Disasters for Your Area

Disasters can strike anywhere, yet certain locations face greater vulnerability to particular catastrophes than others. Many countries, including the US, have online databases that can enlighten you on potential future disasters for your area. In America, we have the Federal Emergency Management Agency (FEMA), the Emergency Alert System (FCC), and the National Oceanic and Atmospheric Administration's National Weather Service (NWS). These agencies collaborate to warn people against approaching severe weather or natural disasters (*The Emergency Alert System (EAS)*, n.d.). Since your apothecary may also cover disasters, it's important to know the sicknesses you may deal with during such emergencies.

Gathering and Organizing Herbs

So, what comes next after mapping out diseases and their herbal cures?

Gathering medicines! Gathering medicines is the focal point of this section. I've already discussed over 90 herbs and what they cure in Chapter 3. I've also covered collecting herbs and preparing them in Chapter 4. Now, you'll learn how to organize them. Organizing medicines is easy compared to all the practical steps we have discussed already. But without doing it properly, you won't feel good about yourself when the need arises to use an herbal remedy, and you can't find it despite knowing it's there somewhere.

The Environment for Herbs

Building an apothecary typically takes time, as collecting the necessary items is a gradual process. However, organizing a high-quality apothecary is a straightforward task once the collection is gathered. Situate the apothecary in a cool, dry place, away from sunlight. The reason is that moisture, light, and air can reduce the potency of herbs. I talked about this under packaging in Chapter 4. Any stored medicine that moisture can reach will start to decompose over time. Powders would compact. As such, your containers should be lightproof and airproof because moisture travels in the air. This is why droplets appear on the bottle of your ice-cold drink, even when the air feels extremely dry.

The Containers for Herbs

Containers for your herbs in a natural medicine apothecary should prioritize functionality and preservation. Opt for airtight jars or containers that shield the herbs from light and moisture, maintaining their potency for longer durations.

Protecting from light is the reason companies make tincture bottles opaque. I don't advise putting alcoholic tinctures in plastic bottles due to chemical reactions between alcohol and other plastics. Herbal bottles, tins, and jars are specifically designed for such liquids and other concoctions, or at least you can preserve them in there (*Cannabis Dropper Bottle Packaging*, n.d.).

Containers you can use for storing herbs in an apothecary include:

- airproof jars, tins, and bottles

- airtight paper bags

- airproof sacks

- dropper bottles

- nursing bottles

- nylon and plastic bags

- freezer

- cupboard

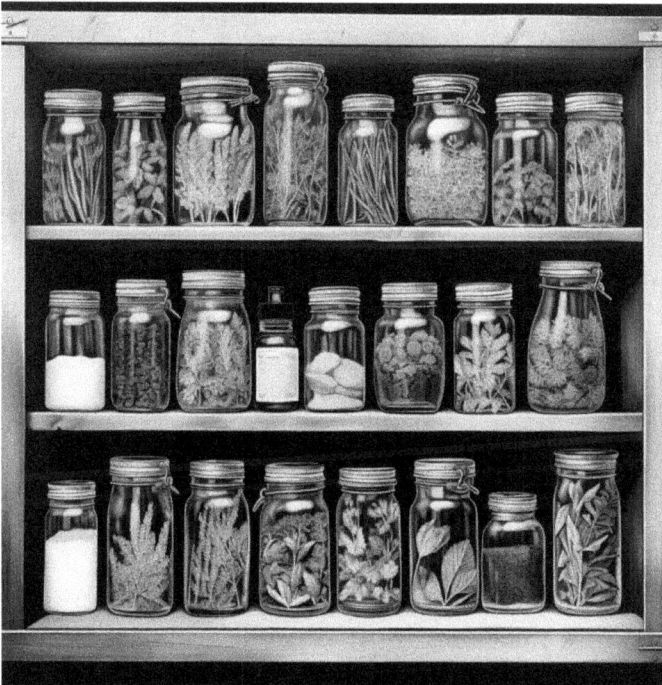

You can freeze fresh herbs safely for 8–12 weeks (Burton-Hughes, 2019). If you don't want to freeze them, immerse them in water in an airtight container. Alternatively, soak a paper towel and wrap the fresh herbs in it before putting it inside an airproof container. They'll last longer in there than out of the container but less than when you freeze them (Domrongchai, 2023).

You also need the following equipment for a complete apothecary:

- Fine mesh sieve

- Mortar and pestle

- Funnels

- Kitchen scale

- Teapot

- Dropper bottle

Fine Mesh Sieve

Various sieves of different sizes are necessary for straining herbal products such as tea, tinctures, and infused oil. However, in my experience, a potato ricer is more effective when filtering a substantial quantity of tincture. Its capability to strain the biomass ensures the extraction of even a single drop of liquid. Sieves aren't great for such tasks as the downward pressure can damage them. But if you don't intend to strain the biomass, a less sturdy sieve would do.

Cheesecloth

Cheesecloth is best for filtering the tincture you intend to strain. To buy the best cheesecloth, look for one made of cotton and without bleach (Mason, n.d.). Otherwise, some filtrates will be altered chemically from the reaction with bleach. I think this is a must-have material for anyone who intends to use tinctures a lot.

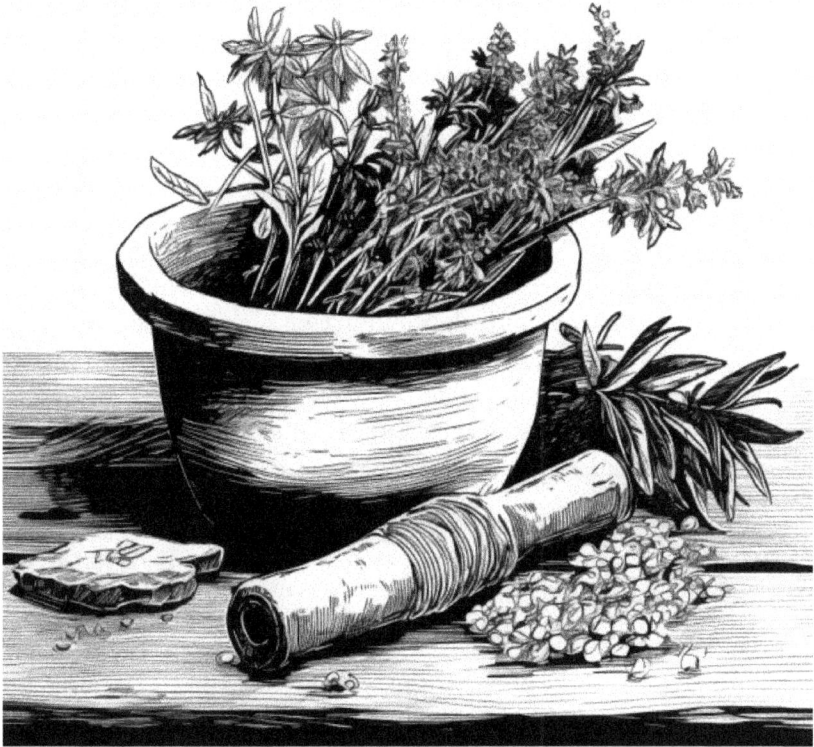

A mortar and pestle is more convenient for grinding an assortment of herbs. The set is more reliable than an electric or handheld grinder since it doesn't easily get spoiled, and anyone can use it without any prior operational knowledge. However, the advanced grinders are faster and demand less work.

Unless absolutely necessary, I don't like grinding herbs before storage. It's better to grind it when you need to use it. Herbal powders oxidate, meaning some compounds escape into the air, which reduces their potency. Storing the herb whole prevents this undesirable phenomenon.

Funnels

Your apothecary should contain funnels for transferring liquids between containers. Even with adept pouring skills, spillage is inevitable, resulting in both wastage and a messy situation. Crafting certain herbal remedies can prove challenging, limiting their quantity. However, with the appropriate funnel, you can retain every precious drop, ensuring minimal waste and maximum yield, especially for intricate formulations.

Kitchen Scale

Some herbs require precise measurement, especially when giving them to kids. Kava is such an herb. It shouldn't be given to kids because of the strong intoxicating effects it produces and the potential risks to liver health. A kitchen scale will enable you to take the amount you want— no more, no less. Graduated cups are also helpful for precise dosing, especially with liquids.

Teapot

While teapots and tea strainers might seem redundant when you possess an array of pots and sieves, they offer unmatched convenience, specifically tailored for tea preparation. Their functionality is not only advantageous but also more fitting for the task at hand. (Dana, 2019).

Dropper Bottle

A dropper bottle serves as an essential tool for effectively applying herbal remedies meant for ear and eye concerns. Certain herbal blends are specifically designed to address issues related to these sensitive areas. Utilizing dropper bottles not only simplifies the application process but also ensures precise dosage. While it might seem like an easily accessible item, in unforeseen circumstances where access to shops or supplies is limited, obtaining these bottles can become unexpectedly challenging. Hence, it's prudent to have them on hand, even if you are not currently experiencing ear or eye issues, to be prepared for potential emergencies.

Arranging the Containers

Optimize the organization of your apothecary by arranging its contents alphabetically. This simple yet effective system minimizes the time spent searching for specific items. Additionally, maintaining a consistently clean environment within the apothecary is crucial. A pristine setting instills confidence, ensuring both yourself and others feel assured about utilizing the medicines stored within.

The Herbal First Aid

An herbal first-aid kit is a mini, portable version of your apothecary. Its setup should mimic the conventional one in function and organization. Accidents and sudden health emergencies require immediate attention. In the event of a disaster, individuals might experience dislocated joints, fractured or broken bones, and severe burns. Additionally, cuts or punctures, often caused by contaminated or rusty objects, can pose serious health risks. You may stop the bleeding by pressing down on the wound with a clean cloth. But what do you do after the bleeding stops?

This open wound is susceptible to infection if left untreated. This is precisely where your antibacterial ointments and healing gels prove invaluable. I described several herbs with such properties in Chapter 3. We've realized that any herb holds the potential to be crafted into either a solid or liquid remedy. By blending oil infusions with beeswax, we can create gels or ointments that effectively eliminate bacteria from wounds and serve as a preventive measure.

Fractures and Broken Bones

If you have the expertise to splint fractures and mend broken bones, it's essential to complement these skills with herbal remedies for pain relief, like arnica or willow bark, and formulations that effectively reduce swelling, such as turmeric or ginger. These natural remedies serve as invaluable complements, ensuring comprehensive care and comfort for those in need of immediate assistance. Finally, some herbal remedies should be able to heal and prevent bacterial infections. You can make a custom herbal mix comprising different herbs with antibacterial and anti-inflammation properties. It can be an ointment, gel, or wound wash.

Heart Attack First Aid

A heart attack can kill within 24 hours. Doctors say anyone who suffers a sudden heart attack should chew and swallow aspirin provided they aren't allergic to or advised against taking it. This recommendation closely follows aspirin's anti-blood-clotting feature, which helps minimize damage to the heart. The herbal substitutes for aspirin are ginger, turmeric, and a few other herbs. They also prevent blood clotting (Ruggeri, 2021).

If you want a first-aid solution for heart attacks in your apothecary, consider keeping ginger tinctures or rhizomes. The rule of thumb in herbal first aid is to make a list of common sicknesses that can kill within hours or days. Find out the medicines doctors recommend for such diseases and look for their herbal alternatives (that have the same effect). Gradually, you'd build a complete herbal first aid ready for any health emergencies. Some diseases that can kill within hours include cerebrovascular disease, lower respiratory infections, tuberculosis, chronic obstructive pulmonary disease, lung cancer, diarrhea, HIV/Aids, and others (Mayo Clinic, 2018).

Adopting Herbalism In Your Life

To harness the true power of herbs, grasp the philosophy and principles of herbalism and integrate them into your lifestyle. Central to herbalists' beliefs is the interconnectedness of everything, especially concerning health. They view the world as a vast mechanism where every component has a role. Similarly, the human body operates like a finely tuned machine, each part contributing to specific functions. Herbalists emphasize that our well-being relies on the harmony of internal and external systems. If one aspect falters, it disrupts the whole system, impacting overall health.

Immunity and Our Environment and Activities

When a part of the body isn't working properly, it shows a disturbance in the intricate health system, affecting how the body functions. This might mean the body neglects necessary actions, does things it shouldn't, consumes the wrong substances, or misses essential nutrients. These disruptions upset the balance crucial for overall well-being.

One might also encounter harmful substances or stimuli through inhalation, hearing, sight, ingestion, or touch. Examples encompass exposure to loud noises, such as those from acoustic weapons, flash burns caused by welding machines, physical harm from contact, imbalanced diets—excessive sugar or insufficient fiber intake—lack of exercise, excessive weightlifting, and similar factors.

Given their interconnectedness or direct impact on our health system, any irregular interaction with these factors leads to complications. This notion aligns with the herbalists' belief that everything within our health ecosystem is interlinked and mutually influenced by one another.

Dealing With Unsafe Interactions

The dynamics of this interconnected relationship occasionally fall out of sync. No one remains exempt from this inevitability. It's wiser to bolster the immune system in readiness for these occurrences. This is why herbalism focuses on the holistic treatment and prevention of diseases. Plants contain compounds that work in synergy to maintain them. Certain compounds build the leaves; others extend the roots; others strengthen the stem, and so on. These compounds only work properly with the support of the others. Once herbalists realize a plant substance cures specific diseases, they reason that other substances exist that support the medicinal one. So, instead of isolating that specific substance as Big Pharma does, they'd rather feed you whole plant parts with all their compounds for a holistic treatment.

Herbalists aren't for quick healing like conventional therapy, which glorifies hero medicines. Big Pharma drugs are called hero medicines for their quick impact on compromised immune system nodes with visible symptoms. Herbal compounds thrive on mutual support. When herbalists identify a plant substance with healing properties, they seek others that complement it. Unlike pharmaceutical practices of isolating specific compounds, herbalists advocate for holistic treatments, preferring to utilize whole plant parts along with their various compounds for comprehensive healing. It extends its reach to hidden areas, revealing underlying health issues. Following therapy, both symptoms and root causes tend to vanish.

Sicknesses Have an External Cause

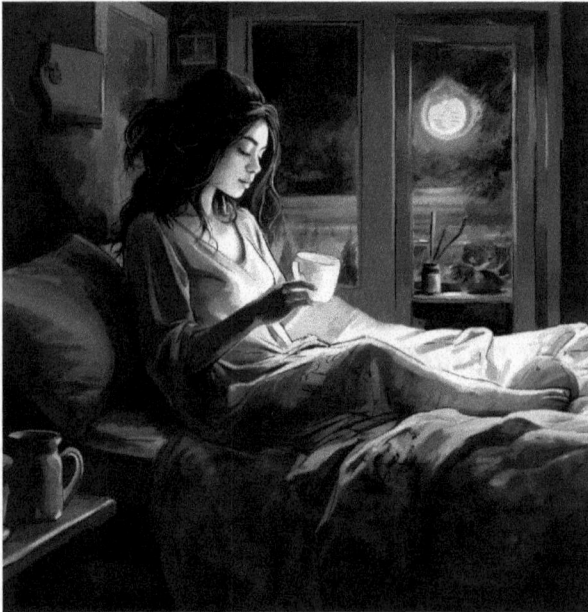

I said before that a person cannot live for years without the balance, relationship, or connection between his immune system and the environment developing problems. Every sickness in the human body can be traced back to an external source. Diabetes comes from excess sugar, and sugar doesn't originate from the body. Hemorrhoids are caused by constipation, unhealthy diets, dehydration, and a sedentary lifestyle. All four factors are external. The detailed explanation of the connection between our immune system and the environment has a specific purpose. It's meant to highlight the importance of understanding and embracing herbalism properly. Symptoms often appear when the immune system is compromised, and not all these issues can be detected through routine medical tests (Herbal, 2018).

Herbalism's Health Doctrine

Herbalism aims to address undiscovered health gaps by taking a holistic approach. Continuing with the hemorrhoids example, to treat it the idea is to incorporate anti-constipation herbs and aids that promote digestion into your routine. This includes adequate hydration, a fiber-rich diet, and regular exercise. Following this regimen could potentially alleviate hemorrhoids for good. Unlike medical procedures, which might not offer a lasting solution, the herbal method outlined here provides a more sustainable approach to treating piles.

Therefore, herbalism cures and prevents. Conventional medicines only cure. This is why herbalists make select herbs a part of their regular diet. Becoming a true herbalist requires forging a deep connection with your hero herbs, which you can only discover by trying a range of plant-based solutions (Popham, 2017). But remember to coordinate with a qualified doctor while transitioning from conventional to herbal medicine. Start with small doses and increase them accordingly when your body adapts.

Conclusion

When it comes to crafting your herbal first aid kit, I've provided you with a versatile guide adaptable to any scale you need. Crafting a natural first-aid kit calls for ingenuity. Start by understanding the contents and functions of traditional first-aid kits before fashioning their herbal counterparts. Often, the more commonly used herbal first-aid items will make their way into your main first-aid kit! It's okay to have these natural medicine options in multiple spots for use when your family may need them most.

Ensure that your kit covers any prevalent familial health conditions that could lead to sudden emergencies. Transitioning to herbal healing is a gradual journey, often spanning months or even years, particularly if your body is accustomed to conventional medications. Alongside exploring herbalism, prioritize regular exercise and a nourishing diet. If you're currently on medication or managing a specific illness, involve a medical professional in the transition process for guidance and support.

Conclusion

Throughout "Natural Medicine and Herbal Remedies for Preppers: Survival Secrets of Wilderness Wellness," you've traversed the landscape of preparedness. Now equipped with the wisdom to establish an herbal apothecary and a natural first aid kit, you've fortified your family's well-being against even the most formidable challenges. Your commitment echoes loud and clear: never again caught unprepared, ensuring your loved ones thrive amidst the unpredictable trials of life.

Cultivating and crafting herbs feels more like a joy than a task, not just for me but for many herbalists. The world of herbalism offers a straightforward path to mastery and practice. Whether foraging, tending to gardens, preparing remedies, or storing herbs, I find immense satisfaction in every step. As you've made it this far in the book, my hope is this sparks a similar feeling in you! Engaging in herbalism fosters a sense of mindfulness toward one's health while simultaneously erasing the fear of ailments.

Exploring past disasters unveils the health hurdles individuals encountered, offering invaluable insights to proactively prepare for future crises. This lets you prepare for disasters accordingly. Pay special attention to the warning signs and the resulting hardships like diseases, starvation, violence, social disorder, and more. All these need unique prepping.

While reading about plant medicines online, you'll likely bump into articles that seek to discourage their use. Instead of guiding towards safe use, they emphasize the risks and even narrate stories of people who died or suffered serious injuries after taking certain herbs. This saps your enthusiasm and confidence about herbs. Unless you are armed with sufficient knowledge of herbal history, particularly its effectiveness, and you are aware of the scientific and logical arguments for it, these articles may prove deadly for your herbal zeal for good. Hence, I dedicated significant time to thorough research, aiming to dispel the apprehensions sowed by the pessimistic voices on the internet regarding herbal remedies.

You want to know as many herbs as possible, with special emphasis on their uses, side effects, dosage, and who can or cannot use them. This book dissects 92 herbs and covers almost all the popular ones in America today. The wisdom behind learning about many herbs is to gain the ability to create or invent strong herbal concoctions, easily identify substitutes, and deal with different diseases.

But knowing many herbs offers little advantage if you can't get them. Buying, foraging, and especially farming are important and probably necessary for true herbalism. Growing them puts you in total control of quality, quantity, and form (fresh vs. dried). However, even herbal gardeners must sometimes purchase the stuff since it can be tough to nurture 500 different herbs in a small garden. Diversifying your sources for herbs is the surest way to get everything you need.

To get the most from herbs, it is important to master the philosophies and principles upon which herbalists operate. Chief among these are the concepts of holistic medicine, naturalism, and optimal health. Holistic medicine advocates two things regarding therapy: Using whole plant parts as opposed to isolated compounds and treating the whole body instead of specific parts. Naturalism promotes the use of natural medicine not synthesized in a lab. Optimizing health is the primary goal of herbalism. Fight diseases before they afflict you. That doesn't mean taking preventive synthesized drugs, which may have side effects, high costs, and a bad smell or taste. But it means making food your medicine, and medicine your food.

In most cases, you must couple herbal therapy with lifestyle changes for the best results. So, while incorporating herbs into your lifestyle, your target should be health optimization, holistic treatment, and green remedies. Involve a doctor in your mission to transition from pharmaceutical to herbal therapy, especially if you have an underlying disease or are undergoing treatment. Not consulting doctors and herbalism experts exposes you to certain risks that can be costly. You can talk to me anytime if you need help with your herbal explorations.

As you conclude this book, embrace its principles as companions on your journey to a more secure future. Let these teachings become a legacy, guiding not just you but your loved ones. May the wisdom of herbal remedies, natural medicine, and self-sufficiency fortify you all. With this knowledge, together, you're equipped for any hurdle and empowered to flourish in any circumstance, ensuring a resilient path ahead for generations.

Stay prepared friends!

As an independent author with a small marketing budget, reviews are my livelihood on this platform. I would be incredibly thankful if you could take just 60 seconds to write a brief review on Amazon, even if it's just a few sentences!

You can do so by scanning the QR code taking you to my author page on Amazon. Find this book to review, or shop for other best-sellers in my prepping collection! I do love hearing from my readers, and I personally read every single review. Thank you for the support!

Leave a 1-Click Review!

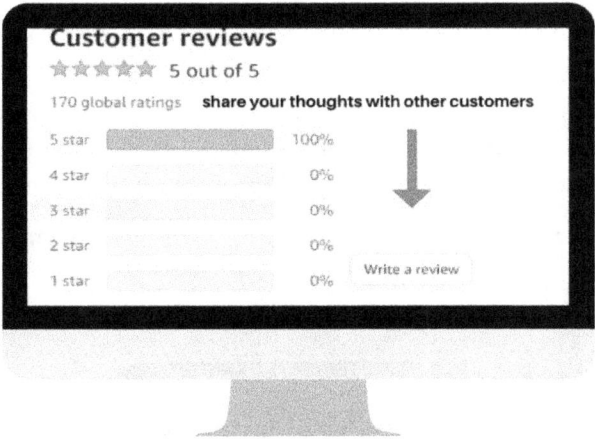

Customer reviews

★★★★★ 5 out of 5

170 global ratings   **share your thoughts with other customers**

5 star		100%
4 star		0%
3 star		0%
2 star		0%
1 star		0%

Write a review

Scan the QR code below

SCAN ME

EXTRA BONUS

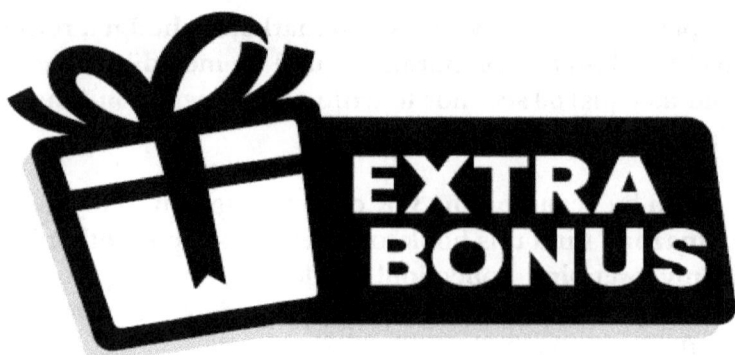

Thank you for embarking on this literary journey with me! Your support and enthusiasm for my book mean the world. As a token of gratitude, I'm thrilled to offer you exclusive access to the "Herbal Medicine Starter Guide." Simply scan the QR code below and drop your email to receive this invaluable tool – no strings attached, just a little something extra for being a loyal reader. Your continued support is truly appreciated, and I hope this bonus enriches your prepping journey in the most extraordinary ways!

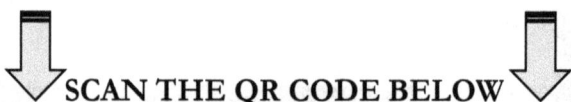

⬇ SCAN THE QR CODE BELOW ⬇

SCAN ME

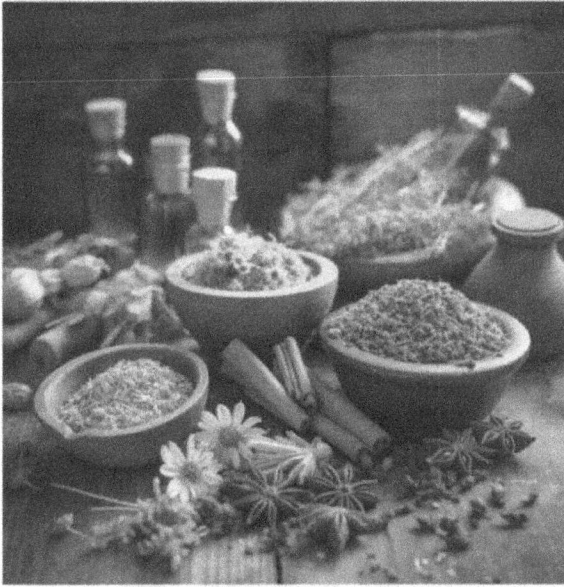

GLOSSARY OF HERBS

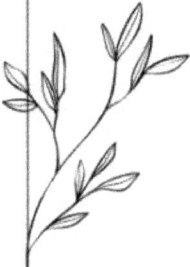

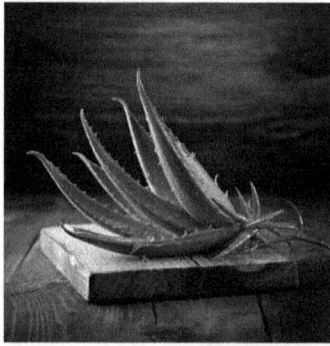

Aloe Vera: A succulent plant known for its soothing and healing properties for the skin.

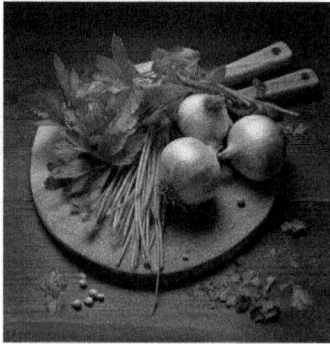

Amla (Gooseberry): A fruit known for its high vitamin C content and medicinal properties.

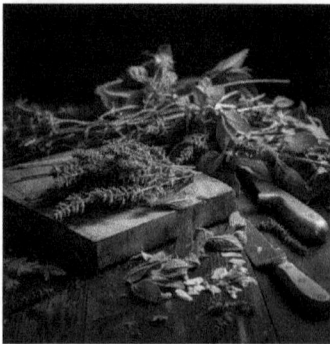

American Skullcap: A herb used for its potential calming and anti-anxiety effects.

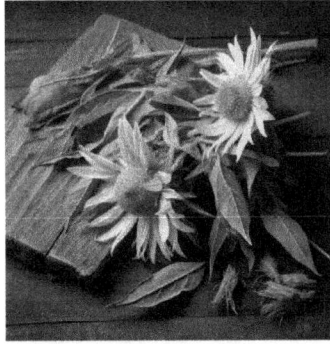

Arnica: A flowering plant used for its anti- inflammatory and pain-relieving properties.

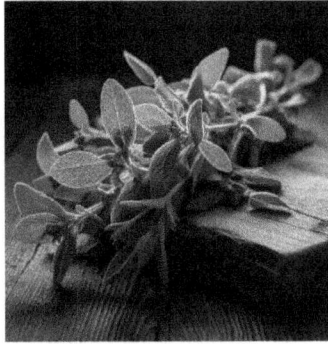

Ashwagandha: An adaptogenic herb used for stress relief and overall wellness.

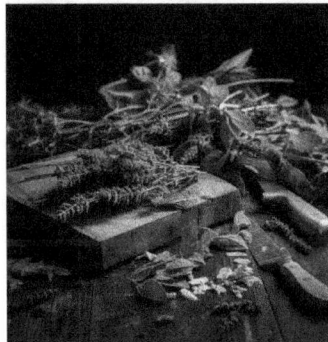

Astragalus: A herb known for its immune- boosting properties.

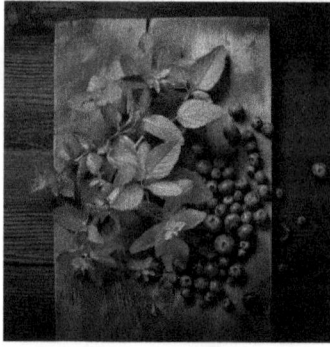

Bilberry: A fruit rich in antioxidants, often used for eye health.

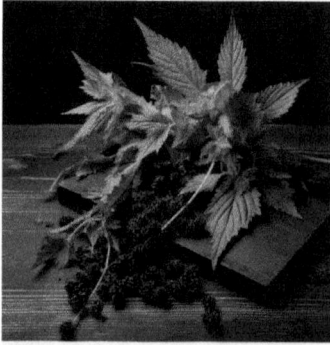

Black Cohosh: A herb commonly used for menopausal symptoms.

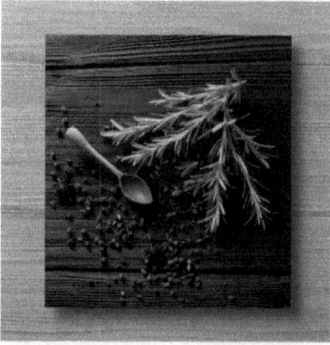

Black Cumin: Seeds known for their potential health benefits, including immune support.

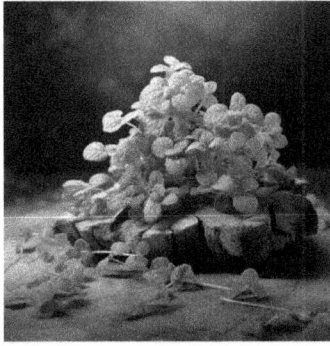

Brahmi: An herb used in traditional medicine for cognitive health.

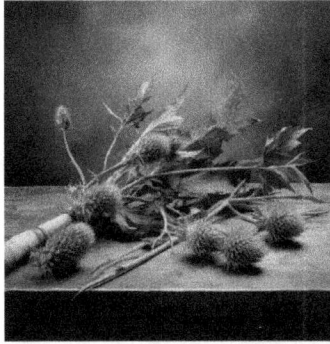

Burdock: A plant with roots used for various health purposes, including detoxification.

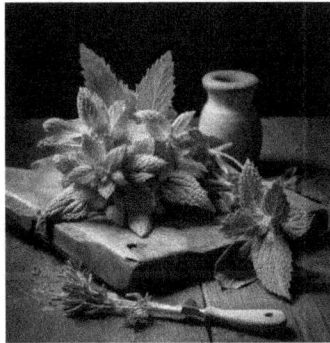

Butterbur: A plant used historically for migraines and allergy relief.

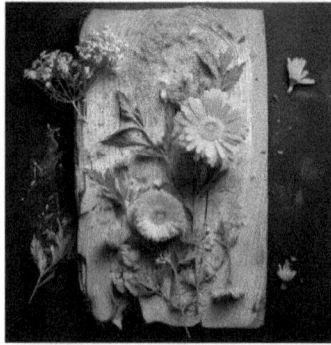

Calendula: A flower known for its anti- inflammatory and skin-soothing properties.

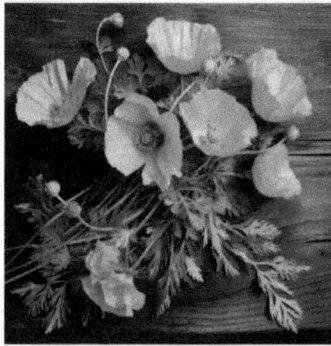

California Poppy: A plant used for relaxation and possible pain relief.

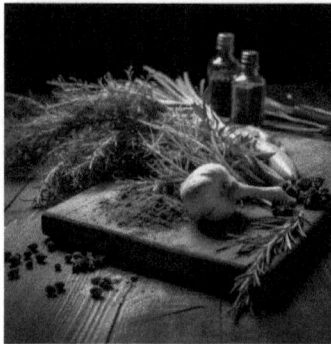

Caraway: Seeds used for digestive health and flavoring.

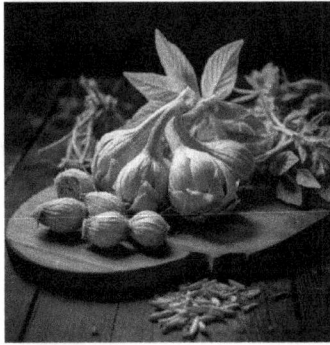

Cardamom: Seeds or pods used for flavoring and potential health benefits.

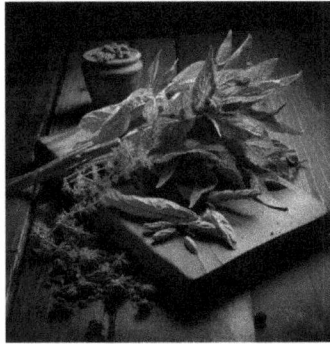

Cat's Claw: A vine traditionally used in herbal medicine for various ailments.

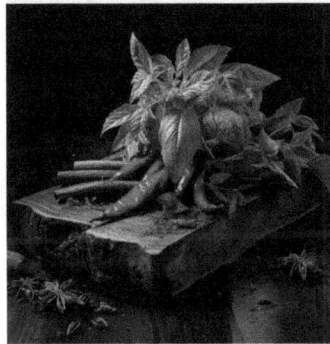

Cayenne: A spice known for its potential health benefits, including pain relief.

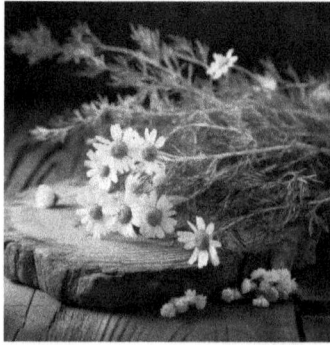

Chamomile: A flower often used for its calming and sleep-inducing properties.

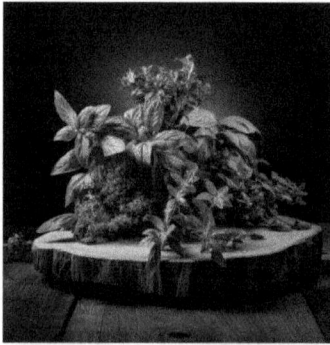

Chaste Tree: A plant often used for hormonal balance in women.

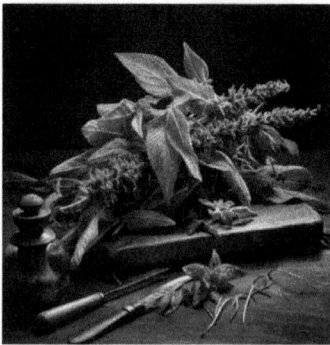

Chinese Skullcap: An herb used in traditional Chinese medicine for various purposes.

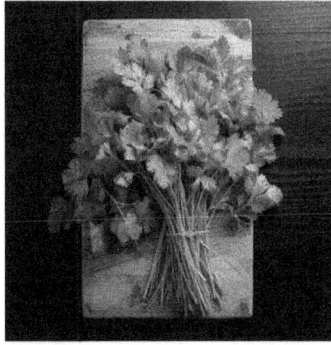

Cilantro: An herb used in cooking and traditional medicine for its flavor and potential health benefits.

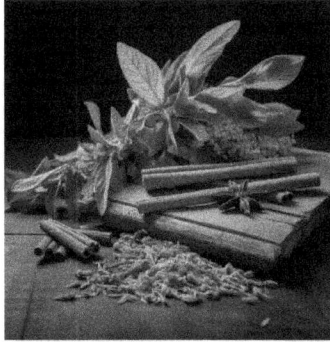

Cinnamon: A spice known for its flavor and potential health-promoting properties.

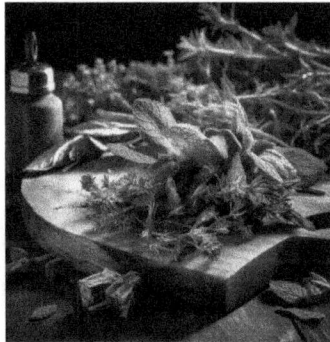

Cleavers: A plant historically used for its diuretic properties.

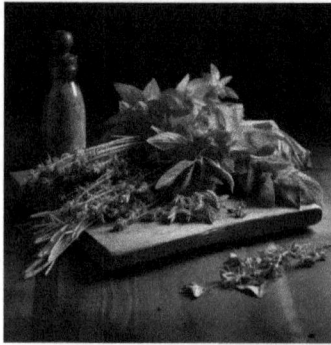

Codonopsis or Dangshen: An herb used in traditional Chinese medicine for energy and immunity.

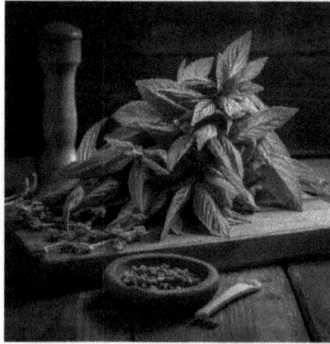

Comfrey: A plant known for its potential healing properties, though internal use is cautioned.

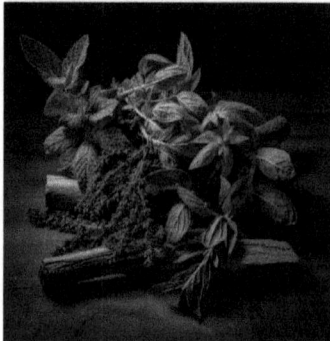

Cramp Bark: A plant historically used for menstrual and muscle cramp relief.

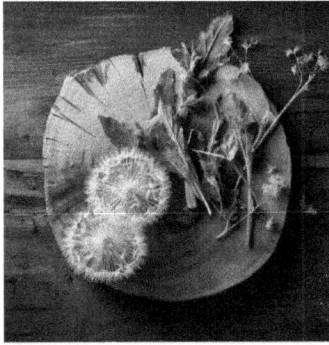

Dandelion: A plant whose leaves and roots are used for various health purposes.

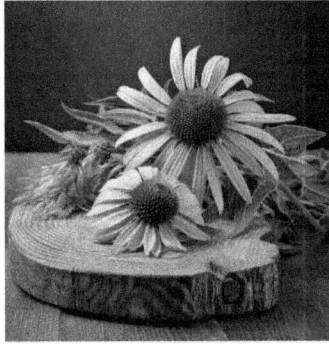

Echinacea: A herb often used for immune support.

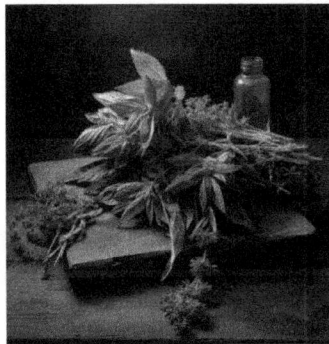

Elder: A plant with flowers and berries used in traditional medicine.

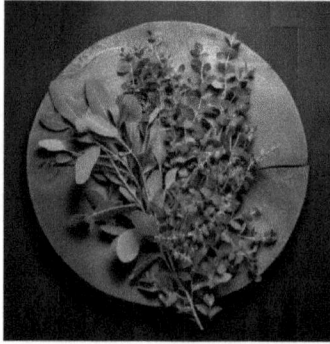

Eucalyptus: A tree known for its essential oil used for respiratory health.

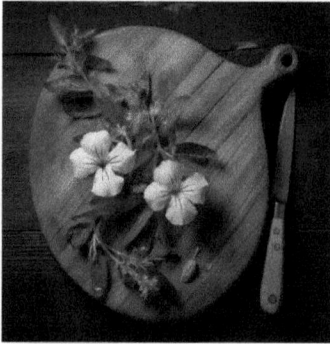

Evening Primrose: A plant known for its oil used in skincare and potential health benefits.

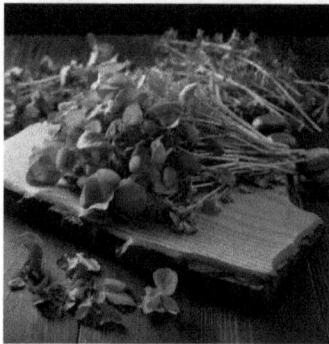

Fenugreek: Seeds used in cooking and traditional medicine for various purposes.

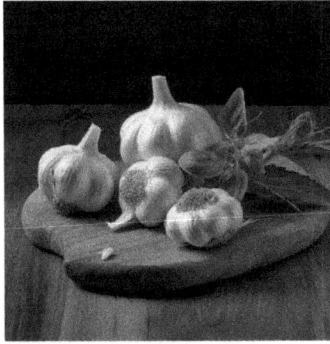

Garlic: A bulb used in cooking and traditional medicine for its potential health benefits.

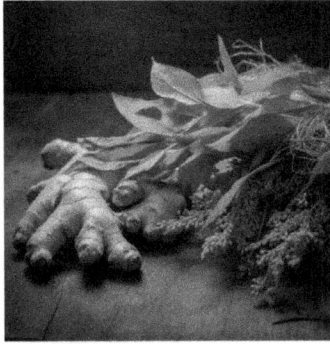

Ginger: A root used in cooking and traditional medicine for its digestive and anti-inflammatory properties.

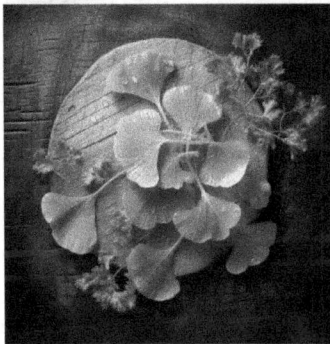

Ginkgo Biloba: An herb known for potential cognitive and circulatory benefits.

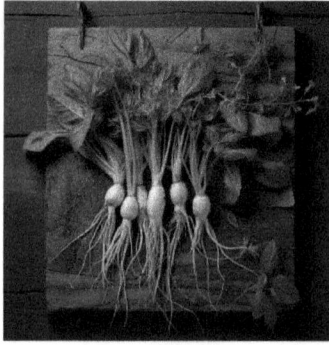

Ginseng: A root used in traditional medicine for energy and overall wellness.

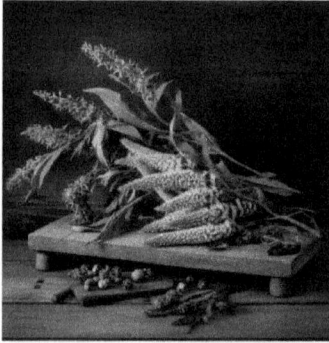

Goldenrod: A plant traditionally used for urinary tract health.

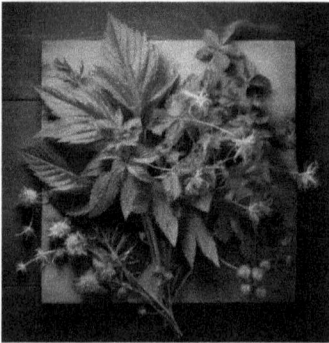

Goldenseal: A herb known for its potential antibacterial properties.

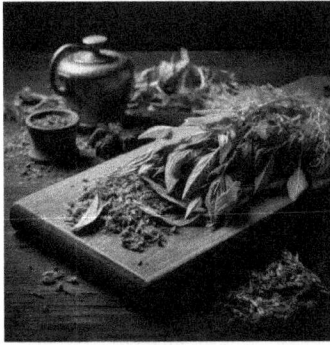

Green Tea: Tea made from unfermented leaves, known for its antioxidants and potential health benefits.

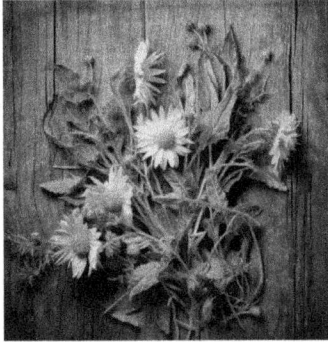

Grindelia: A plant used historically for respiratory issues.

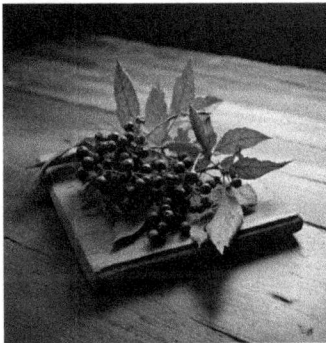

Guarana: A plant whose seeds are used for their stimulant properties.

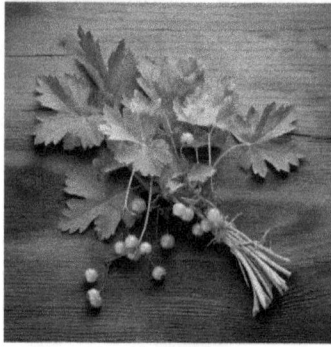

Hawthorn: A plant known for potential heart health benefits.

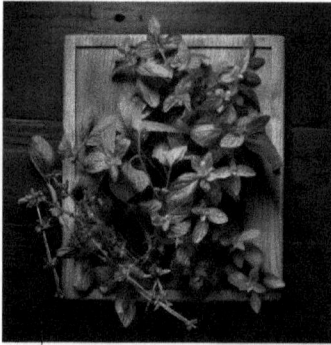

Honeysuckle: A flower used in traditional medicine for its potential anti-inflammatory properties.

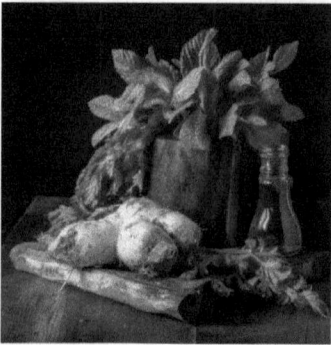

Horseradish: A root used in cooking and traditional medicine for its pungent flavor and potential health benefits.

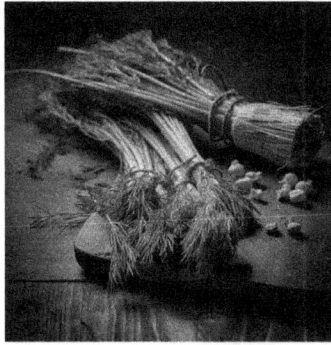

Horsetail: A plant known for its potential diuretic properties.

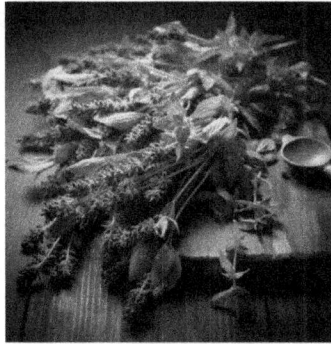

Hyssop: A herb historically used for respiratory and digestive issues.

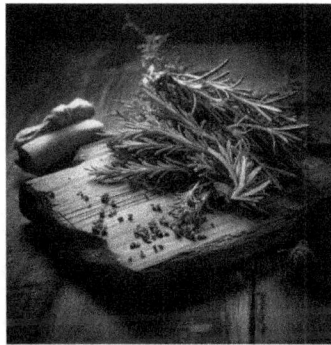

Juniper: Plant whose berries are used for their potential diuretic and digestive properties.

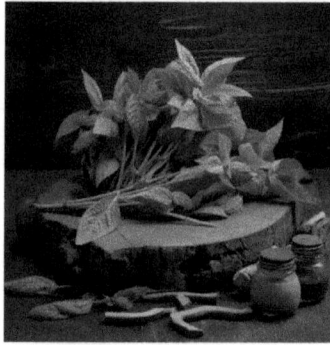

Kava Kava: A plant used for its potential calming effects.

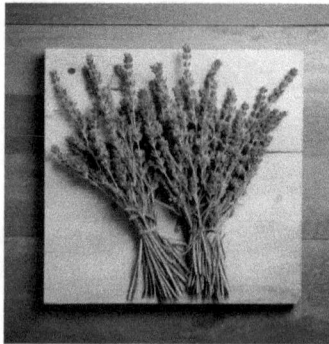

Lavender: Flower known for its calming and aromatherapy properties.

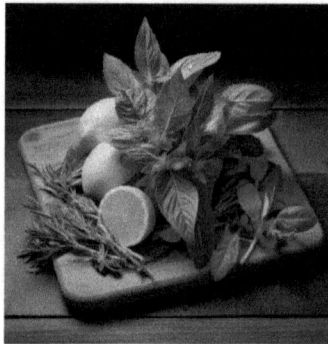

Lemon Balm: Herb known for its calming effects and potential benefits for mood.

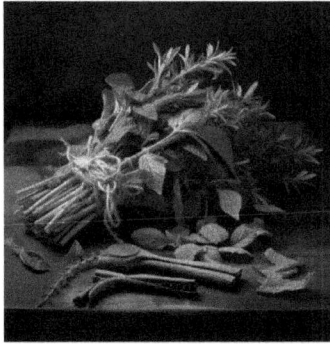

Licorice Root: Root used in traditional medicine for its potential digestive and respiratory benefits.

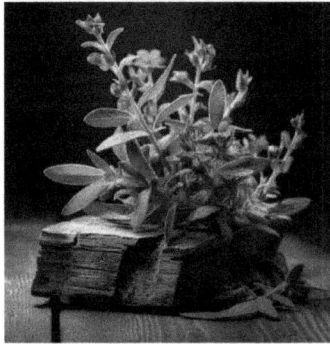

Lobelia: Plant historically used for respiratory issues, but caution is advised due to toxicity.

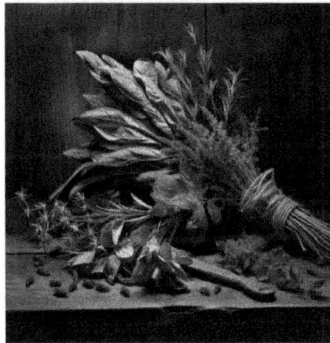

Ma Huang: An herb historically used for respiratory issues, containing ephedrine, with potential side effects.

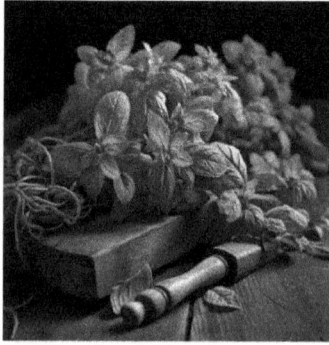

Marjoram: An herb used in cooking and traditional medicine for its flavor and potential health benefits.

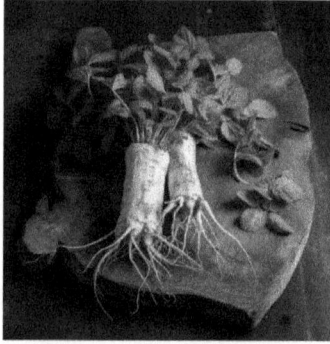

Marshmallow Root: A root used for its potential soothing properties, particularly for the throat and digestive tract.

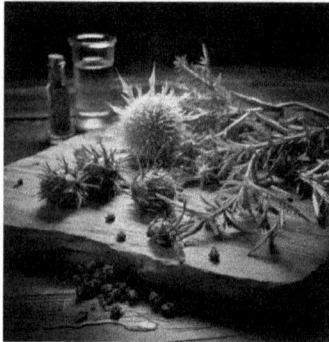

Milk Thistle: A plant known for potential liver health benefits.

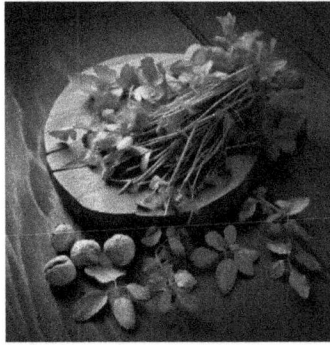

Moringa: A plant known for its nutritional value and potential health benefits.

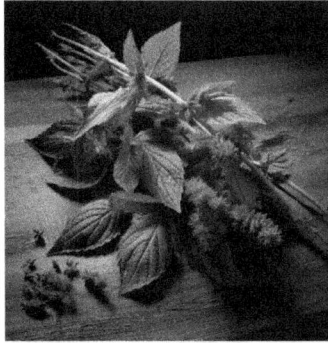

Motherwort: A plant historically used for menstrual issues and potential calming effects.

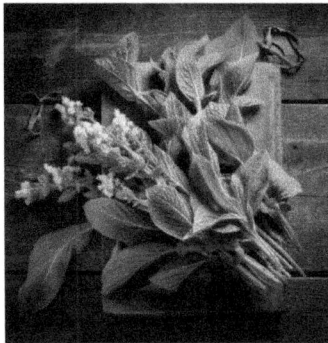

Mullein: A plant whose leaves are used for respiratory issues.

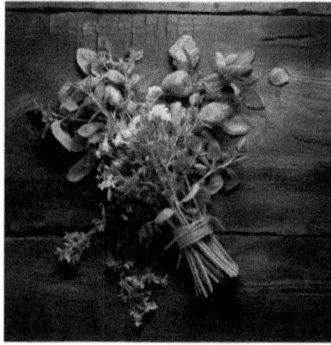

Mustard: Seeds or leaves used in cooking and traditional medicine for various purposes.

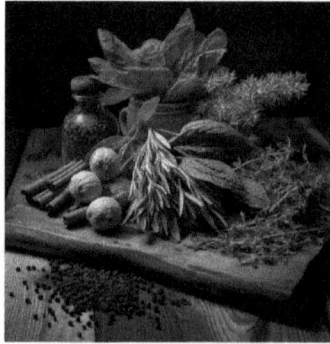

Neem: Tree known for its potential antibacterial and skincare properties.

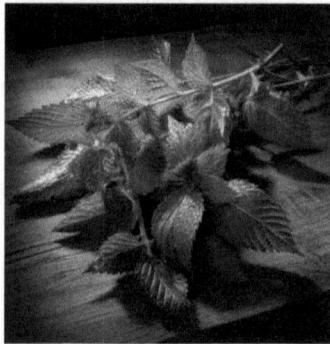

Nettle: Plant used traditionally for its potential anti-inflammatory properties.

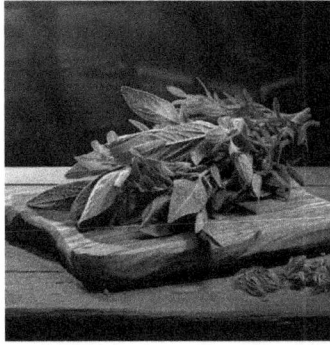

Nutmeg: Spice used in cooking and traditional medicine for flavor and potential health benefits.

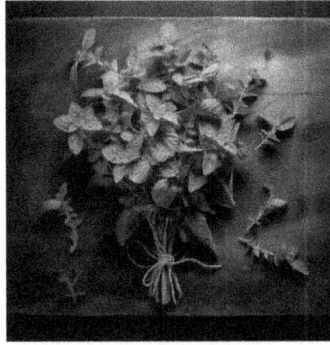

Oregano: An herb used in cooking and traditional medicine for flavor and potential health benefits.

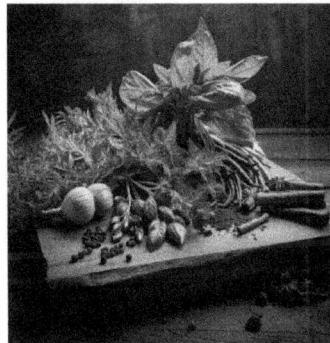

Paprika: Spice made from dried peppers, used for flavoring.

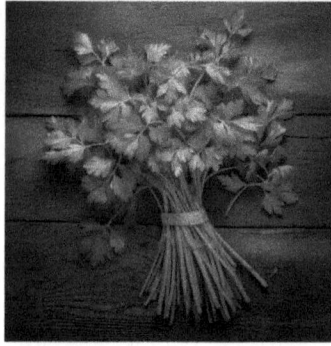

Parsley: An herb used in cooking and traditional medicine for flavor and potential health benefits.

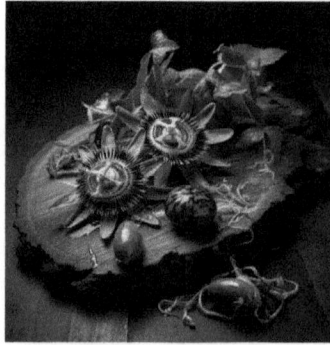

Passionflower: Plant known for its potential calming and sleep-inducing effects.

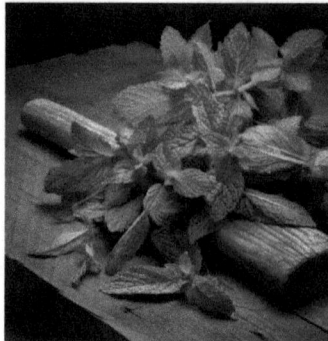

Peppermint: An herb used for its flavor and potential digestive and soothing properties.

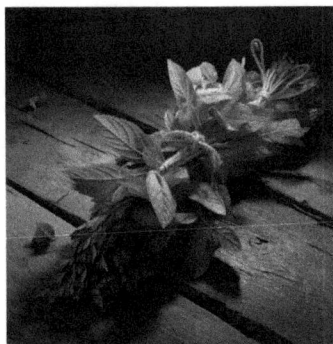

Perilla: A plant used in cooking and traditional medicine, potentially for allergies and digestive issues.

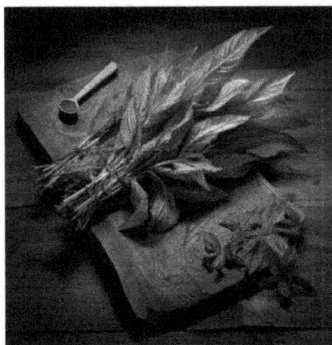

Plantain: A plant known for potential wound- healing and anti-inflammatory properties.

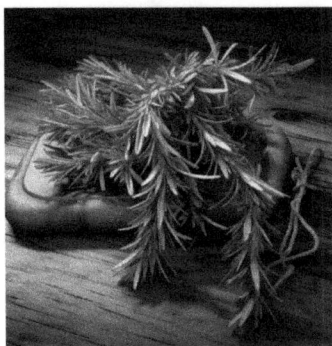

Rosemary: An herb used in cooking and traditional medicine for flavor and potential health benefits.

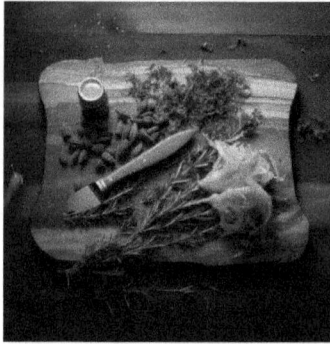

Saffron: A spice derived from flower stigma, used for flavoring and potential health benefits.

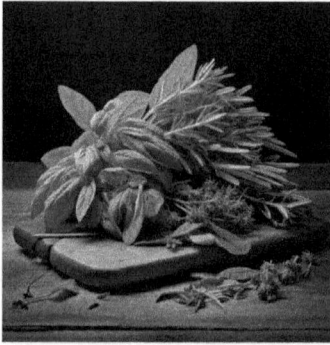

Sage: An herb used in cooking and traditional medicine for flavor and potential health benefits.

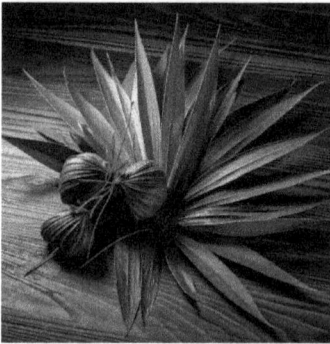

Saw Palmetto: A plant often used for potential prostate health benefits.

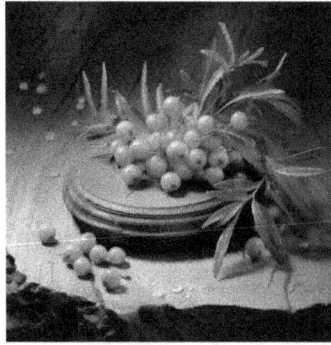

Sea Buckthorn: A plant known for its potential skincare and nutritional benefits.

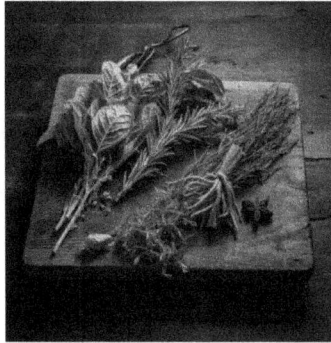

Sida: A plant historically used in traditional medicine for various purposes.

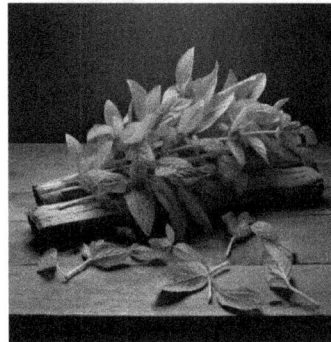

Soy: A legume used in various forms for its nutritional benefits.

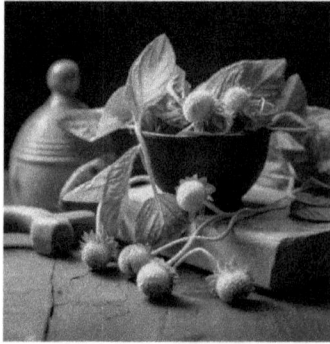

Spilanthes: A plant known for potential oral health benefits.

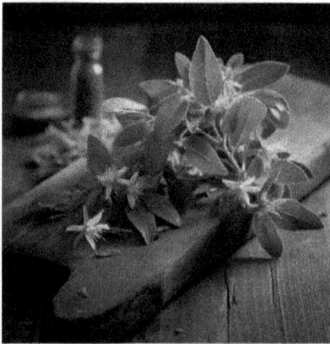

St. John's Wort: A herb used for potential mood-boosting effects.

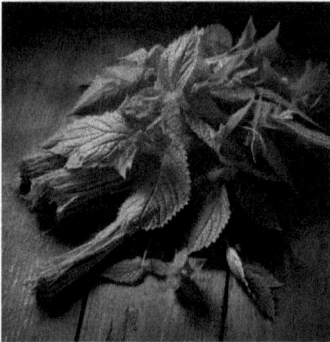

Stinging Nettle: A plant traditionally used for its potential anti-inflammatory properties.

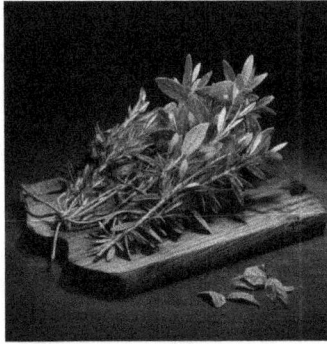

Tarragon: An herb used in cooking, primarily for adding flavoring.

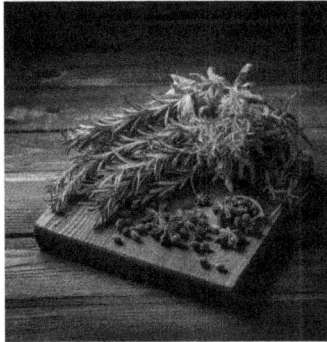

Tea Tree: An essential oil derived from a tree, known for its potential antibacterial properties.

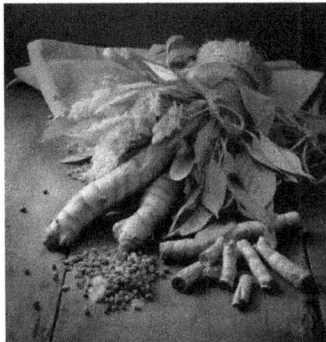

Turmeric: A spice known for its anti- inflammatory and potential health benefits

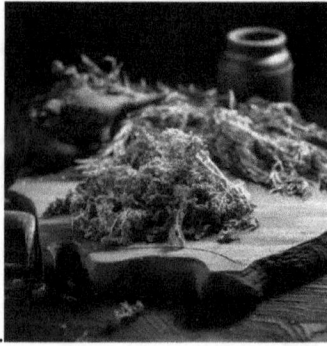

Usnea: A lichen known for potential antibacterial properties.

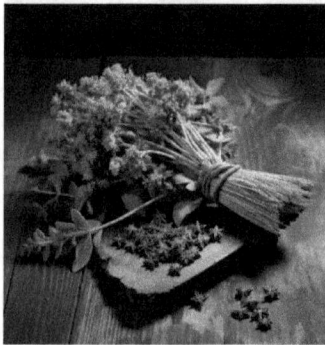

Valerian: A root used for its potential calming and sleep-inducing effects.

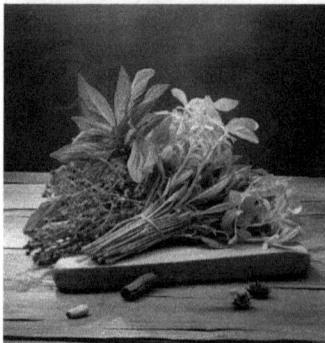

White Willow: Bark known for its potential pain-relieving properties, containing salicin.

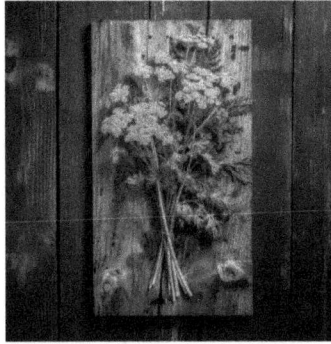

Yarrow: A flowering plant used traditionally for its potential wound-healing properties and to aid in various ailments.

***

Aromatherapy: The use of aromatic plant extracts and essential oils to promote well-being.

Berberine: A compound found in various plants, known for its potential health benefits.

Decoction: Extracting the essence of medicinal plants or herbs by boiling.

Drying: The process of preserving herbs or plants by removing moisture.

Essential Oil: Concentrated oils extracted from plants, often used in aromatherapy or for health purposes.

Infusion: Extracting flavors or medicinal properties by soaking herbs or plants in liquid (usually hot).

Preservation: Techniques used to maintain the quality and properties of herbs or plants for extended use.

Quercetin: A plant compound found in various foods, known for its antioxidant properties.

Remedies: Solutions or treatments used to alleviate or cure health issues.

Tincture: A concentrated herbal extract usually preserved in alcohol.

Wildcrafting: The practice of harvesting plants or herbs from their natural habitat for medicinal or culinary use.

Zinc: A mineral important for various bodily functions, including immune health.

References

A guide to fruit and vegetable production in the Federated States of Micronesia. (n.d.). FAO. https://www.fao.org/3/ca7556en/CA7556EN.pdf

Alam, N. (2023, August 26). *Homemade cornflour/cornstarch recipe.* Cookpad. https://cookpad.com/ng/recipes/15327460-homemade-cornflourcornstarch

Alengebawy, A., Abdelkhalek, S. T., Qureshi, S. R., & Wang, M.-Q. (2021). Heavy Metals and Pesticides Toxicity in Agricultural Soil and Plants: Ecological Risks and Human Health Implications. *Toxics, 9*(3), 42. https://doi.org/10.3390/toxics9030042

Analytical Chemistry. (2018, May 23). Encyclopedia. https://www.encyclopedia.com/science-and-technology/chemistry/chemistry-general/analytical-chemistry#:~:text=Analytical%20chemistry%20began%20in%20the

Briggs, H. (2019, June 11). Plant extinction "bad news for all species." *BBC News.* https://www.bbc.com/news/science-environment-48584515

Buddha quotes. (n.d.). BrainyQuote. https://www.brainyquote.com/quotes/buddha_387356

Burton-Hughes, L. (2019, May 4). *How long does food last in the freezer?* High Speed Training. https://www.highspeedtraining.co.uk/hub/how-long-can-you-store-frozen-food-for/#:~:text=Vegetables%20can%20be%20frozen%20for

Canaway, J. (2019, July 20). *The signs your plants are struggling — and how to rescue them.* ABC Everyday.

https://www.abc.net.au/everyday/signs-your-plant-is-struggling-and-how-to-save-them/11324798

Cannabis Dropper Bottle Packaging. (n.d.). Innovative Packaging Co. https://www.innovativepackagingco.com/tincture-bottles/#:~:text=Tincture%20jars%20or%20bottles%20typically

Cassell, K. (2020). Plants go to war: A botanical history of World War II. *The Yale Journal of Biology and Medicine, 93*(2), 375–379. https://www.ncbi.nlm.nih.gov/pmc/articles/PMC7309670/

Catalysing ancient wisdom and modern science for the health of people and the planet. (2023). World Health Organization . https://www.who.int/initiatives/who-global-centre-for-traditional-medicine

Climate change impacts. (2021, August 13). National Oceanic and Atmospheric Administration. https://www.noaa.gov/education/resource-collections/climate/climate-change-impacts

Climate impacts on human health. (n.d.). United States Environmental Protection Agency. https://climatechange.chicago.gov/climate-impacts/climate-impacts-human-health#:~:text=Warmer%20temperatures%20and%20shifting%20weather

Cody Lundin Quote. (n.d.). A-Z Quotes. Retrieved December 17, 2023, from https://www.azquotes.com/quote/681257

Coulter, L., & Forney, J. M. (n.d.-a). *15 favorite shrubs for shade gardens.* HGTV. Retrieved December 16, 2023, from https://www.hgtv.com/outdoors/flowers-and-plants/trees-and-shrubs/7-shrubs-for-shade-gardens-pictures#:~:text=Luckily%2C%20we%20have%20alternatives%2C%20especially

Coulter, L., & Forney, J. M. (n.d.-b). *15 favorite shrubs for shade gardens.* HGTV. Retrieved December 16, 2023, from https://www.hgtv.com/outdoors/flowers-and-plants/trees-and-shrubs/7-shrubs-for-shade-gardens-pictures#:~:text=Luckily%2C%20we%20have%20alternatives%2C%20especially

CropWatch. (2015, September 17). Ridge Plant. https://cropwatch.unl.edu/tillage/ridge

Dana. (2019, September 5). *10 essential tools every herbalist needs.* Rustic Farm Life. https://www.rusticfarmlife.com/essential-tools-every-herbalist-needs/

Diaz, J. M., & Fridovich-Keil, J. L. (2018). Genetically modified organism. In *Encyclopædia Britannica.* Britannica. https://www.britannica.com/science/genetically-modified-organism

Do you know the signs of a heart attack? (2018). Mayo Clinic. https://www.mayoclinic.org/first-aid/first-aid-heart-attack/basics/art-20056679

Domrongchai, A. (2023, January 9). *Never waste herbs again with these simple tips.* Food & Wine. https://www.foodandwine.com/seasonings/herbs/how-to-store-fresh-herbs#:~:text=Though%20hardier%20herbs%20can%20also

EHA Consulting Group. (n.d.). Food Ingredient Safety. Retrieved December 16, 2023, from https://www.ehagroup.com/food-ingredient-safety/storage-risks/#:~:text=Typically%2C%20time%2C%20temperature%2C%20humidity

Electromagnetic Pulse (EMP): What is EMP and how Is It created? (2003). Washington State Department of Health. https://doh.wa.gov/sites/default/files/legacy/Documents/Pubs/320-090_elecpuls_fs.pdf

18th century book of herbal remedies. (n.d.). Heritage. https://heritage.rcpsg.ac.uk/items/show/187

Encyclopedia. (2018, May 23). Analytical Chemistry. https://www.encyclopedia.com/science-and-technology/chemistry/chemistry-general/analytical-chemistry#:~:text=Analytical%20chemistry%20began%20in%20the

Fabino, A. (2023, October 20). *Doomsday prepping poised to become $2.46 billion industry.* Newsweek. https://www.newsweek.com/doomsday-prepping-246-billion-industry-survival-tools-market-growth-1836530#:~:text=The%20Global%20Survival%20Tools%20Market

Fahey, J. W., Stephenson, K. K., & Wallace, A. J. (2015a). Dietary amelioration of helicobacter infection. *Nutrition Research, 35*(6), 461–473. https://doi.org/10.1016/j.nutres.2015.03.001

Fahey, J. W., Stephenson, K. K., & Wallace, A. J. (2015d). Dietary amelioration of helicobacter infection. *Nutrition Research, 35*(6), 461–473. https://doi.org/10.1016/j.nutres.2015.03.001

Fenton, S., & Ghaddar, A. (2023, October 20). Strait of Hormuz: The world's most important oil artery. *Reuters.* https://www.reuters.com/business/energy/strait-hormuz-worlds-most-important-oil-artery-2023-10-20/

Food processing and nutrition. (2012). Vic.gov.au. https://www.betterhealth.vic.gov.au/health/healthyliving/food-processing-and-nutrition

Garman, A. : J. (2019, February 1). *How to start beekeeping in your backyard.* Backyard Beekeeping. https://backyardbeekeeping.iamcountryside.com/beekeeping-101/how-to-start-a-honey-bee-farm/

Gravalese, S. (2023, July 22). *Dressing for Success: The Importance of Foraging Clothes.* Slow Living Kitchen. https://slowlivingkitchen.com/foraging-clothes/#:~:text=Durable%20and%20Protective%20Outerwear

Gregory, J. (2023, May 15). *Today's biggest threats against the energy grid.* Security Intelligence. https://securityintelligence.com/articles/todays-biggest-threats-against-the-energy-grid/

Gupta, S. (2010). Chamomile: A herbal medicine of the past with a bright future. *Molecular Medicine Reports, 3*(6). https://doi.org/10.3892/mmr.2010.377

Heart disease - symptoms and causes. (n.d.). Mayo Clinic. https://www.mayoclinic.org/diseases-conditions/heart-disease/symptoms-causes/syc-20353118#:~:text=A%20buildup%20of%20fatty%20plaques

Herbal History. (2019). Herbal Academy. https://theherbalacademy.com/herbal-history/

Herbal medicine Information. (n.d.). Mount Sinai Health System. https://www.mountsinai.org/health-library/treatment/herbal-medicine

Herbal, O. W. (2018, May 10). *Principles of home herbalism.* Old Ways Herbal. https://oldwaysherbal.com/2018/05/10/principles-of-home-herbalism/

Huelskoetter, T. (2015, August 20). *Hurricane Katrina's health care legacy.* Center for American Progress. https://www.americanprogress.org/article/hurricane-katrinas-health-care-legacy/#:~:text=The%20storm%20and%20the%20levee

Igbashio, M. D. & O. (2022). Production of local soap using alkali derived from mango and plantain peel. *Journal of Science and Technology Research, 4*(4). https://doi.org/10.5281/zenodo.7395753

Institute of Culinary Education. (2018, November 28). How to Safely Forage. https://www.ice.edu/blog/how-to-safely-forage#:~:text=Don

Joyce Meyer Quotes. (n.d.). BrainyQuote. https://www.brainyquote.com/quotes/joyce_meyer_567639

Karen, S. (2020, June 19). *Where to buy herbs (+ tips to grow your own, too!).* Traditional Cooking School by GNOWFGLINS. https://traditionalcookingschool.com/raising-food/local-food-101-buying-herbs/

Kirk, T. (2022, September 28). Woman killed by herbal remedies she took to treat arthritis. *Evening Standard.* https://www.standard.co.uk/news/uk/herbal-remedies-ayurveda-dangers-medication-inquest-coroner-harrow-b1028686.html

Klinger, J. (2021, June 24). *Top 4 ways to extract essential oils from plants.* Www.customprocessingservices.com. https://www.customprocessingservices.com/blog/top-4-ways-to-extract-essential-oils-from-plants

Kooti, W., Farokhipour, M., Asadzadeh, Z., Ashtary-Larky, D., & Asadi-Samani, M. (2016). The role of medicinal plants in the treatment of diabetes: A systematic review. *Electronic Physician, 8*(1), 1832–1842. https://doi.org/10.19082/1832

Law, R. (2023a, November 3). *Best knives for bushcraft: How to choose a survival knife.* BeaverCraft Tools. https://beavercrafttools.com/blogs/blog/best-knives-for-bushcraft-how-to-choose-a-survival-knife

Law, R. (2023b, November 3). *Best knives for bushcraft: How to choose a survival knife.* BeaverCraft Tools. https://beavercrafttools.com/blogs/blog/best-knives-for-bushcraft-how-to-choose-a-survival-knife

Lee, S., Choi, Y., Jeong, H. S., Lee, J., & Sung, J. (2017). Effect of different cooking methods on the content of vitamins and true retention in selected vegetables. *Food Science and Biotechnology, 27*(2), 333–342. https://doi.org/10.1007/s10068-017-0281-1

Living off-grid — one woman's story. (2021, January 5). Platinum. https://platinum-mag.co.uk/people/living-off-grid-one-womans-story-of-life/

MacMillan, A. (2021, April 7). *Global Warming 101.* NRDC; NRDC. https://www.nrdc.org/stories/global-warming-101#causes

Mason. (n.d.). *Must-Have tools for herbalists.* Mountainroseherbs. https://blog.mountainroseherbs.com/tools-for-herbalists

McKenna, D. (2010). *How long have humans used botanicals?* Taking Charge of Your Health & Wellbeing. https://www.takingcharge.csh.umn.edu/how-long-have-humans-used-botanicals

9 institutions offering herbal medicine courses abroad. (n.d.). Hotcoursesabroad. Retrieved December 14, 2023, from https://www.hotcoursesabroad.com/study/training-degrees/international/herbal-medicine-courses/cgory/pc.7-4/sin/ct/programs.html

Noveille, A. (2021a, June 17). *Best places to buy dried herbs online.* Indie Herbalist. https://blog.indieherbalist.com/places-to-buy-dried-herbs-online/

Noveille, A. (2021b, June 17). *Best places to buy dried herbs online.* Indie Herbalist. https://blog.indieherbalist.com/places-to-buy-dried-herbs-online/

Nworu, C. S., Udeogaranya, P. O., Okafor, C. K., Adikwu, A. O., & Akah, P. A. (2015). Perception, usage and knowledge of herbal medicines by students and academic staff of university of nigeria: A survey. *European Journal of Integrative Medicine, 7*(3), 218–227. https://doi.org/10.1016/j.eujim.2015.01.005

OUPblog. (2015, December 19). *Systemic: Why the world has become a more dangerous place.* OUPblog. https://blog.oup.com/2015/12/systemic-world-global-systems/

Petrovska, B. B. (2012). Historical review of medicinal plants' usage. *Pharmacognosy Reviews, 6*(11), 1. https://doi.org/10.4103/0973-7847.95849

Popham, S. (2017, October 5). *5 ways to deepen your connection to herbs.* The School of Evolutionary Herbalism. https://www.evolutionaryherbalism.com/2017/10/05/5-ways-to-deepen-your-connection-to-herbs/

Pro, E. (2019a, August 26). *The survivalist niche: How preppers are helping grow a multi-billion dollar industry.* Medium. https://ecommercepro.medium.com/the-survivalist-niche-how-preppers-are-helping-grow-a-multi-billion-dollar-industry-8ba0f3d1aad6

Rashrash, M. (2017). Prevalence and predictors of herbal medicine use among adults in the united states. *Journal of Patient Experience, 4*(3), 108–113. https://doi.org/10.1177/2374373517706612

Roots of Western herbalism. (2019). Herbal Academy. https://theherbalacademy.com/herbal-history/

Ruggeri, C. (2021, October 15). *Is it safe to take aspirin every day?* Dr. Axe. https://draxe.com/health/aspirin-side-effects/

Shang, A., Cao, S., Xu, X., Gan, R., Tang, G., Corke, H., Mavumengwana, V., & Li, H. (2019). Bioactive Compounds and Biological Functions of Garlic (Allium sativum L.). *Foods, 8*(7), 246. https://doi.org/10.3390/foods8070246

Strauch, I. (2022, October 22). *Poison Ivy, Poison Oak, and 7 Other Plants That Can Give You a Rash.* Everyday Health. https://www.everydayhealth.com/poison-ivy/rashes-caused-by-poisonous-plants/

Subedi, S., & Sharma, G. N. (2018). The health sector response to the 2015 earthquake in Nepal. *Disaster Medicine and Public Health Preparedness, 12*(4), 543–547. https://doi.org/10.1017/dmp.2017.112

Tabassum, N., & Ahmad, F. (2011). Role of natural herbs in the treatment of hypertension. *Pharmacognosy Reviews, 5*(9), 30–40. https://doi.org/10.4103/0973-7847.79097

The biological weapons threat and nonproliferation options: A survey of senior U.S. decision makers and policy shapers. (2006). In *CARNEGIE ENDOWMENT FOR INTERNATIONAL PEACE* (11–14). https://carnegieendowment.org/files/BIO-survey-final-report.pdf

The Emergency Alert System (EAS). (n.d.). Federal Communications Commission. Retrieved December 16, 2023, from https://www.fcc.gov/emergency-alert-system#:~:text=The%20Federal%20Emergency%20Management%20Agency

The Forager's Toolkit. (2020, June 9). *Essential Equipment and Tools You Need for Wildcrafting*. Eatweeds. https://www.eatweeds.co.uk/toolkit

Toscano, K. (2022, March 28). *Proper plant spacing and why it matters*. Worx Toolshed Blog. https://www.worx.com/blog/proper-plant-spacing-and-why-it-matters/#:~:text=The%20easy%20way%20to%20determine

U.S. military warns against electromagnetic pulse weapons attack. (2018, December 1). Mail Online. https://www.dailymail.co.uk/news/article-6449619/Air-Force-warns-electromagnetic-pulse-weapons-Iran-Russia-North-Korea-destroy-America.html

Vincent, P. (2015). *The EMP threat: The state of preparedness against the threat of a electromagnetic pulse (EMP) event* (p. 1). Committee on Oversight and Accountability. https://oversight.house.gov/wp-content/uploads/2015/05/Pry-Statement-5-13-EMP.pdf

WHO reveals leading causes of death and disability worldwide: 2000-2019. (2020, December 9). World Health Organization. https://www.who.int/news/item/09-12-2020-who-reveals-leading-causes-of-death-and-disability-worldwide-2000-

2019#:~:text=Heart%20disease%20has%20remained%20the%20leading%20cause

Workers' rights during natural disasters. (n.d.). Columbia Southern University. https://www.columbiasouthern.edu/blog/blog-articles/2023/june/workers-rights-during-natural-disasters/

www.ingramcontent.com/pod-product-compliance
Lightning Source LLC
Chambersburg PA
CBHW062130040426
42335CB00039B/1893